'Deeply affecting . . . a testament to the human capacity to draw sustenance from the memories of love, even as those memories are disappearing in the person loved. It is an important book' Kay Redfield Jamison, author of *An Unquiet Mind*

'A detailed account of his decade as a caregiver for his wife, who was diagnosed with early-onset Alzheimer's . . . a poignant memoir that will be useful to caregivers of all ages and occupations' *Kirkus Reviews*

'[Kleinman] reminds us of the moral responsibility to provide care and describes care as the "human glue" which binds together families and communities. Beyond this connection, he contends that individual caregivers can discover purpose, revelation, and gratification in tending to others. Much more than a sad story about suffering, loss, and an inevitably downhill disease, Kleinman's graceful narrative provides the sort of tonic that society sorely needs' *Booklist*

'*The Soul of Care* will leave you shaken but instructed, with an ethical imperative and hopeful lessons regarding how best to cultivate one's humanity over the course of a lifetime' Paul Farmer, MD Harvard Medical School

'Heartfelt, beautifully written, incredibly moving, and so instructive . . . This story will stay with me' Abraham Verghese

'An astute, affecting memoir, candid and prescriptive in equal measure' Stacy Schiff, Pulitzer Prize-winning author

'A poetic, moving, generous, and courageous account. You cannot possibly leave these pages unchanged in your understanding of what real caring means' Don Berwick, Institute for Healthcare Improvement

'At once a manifesto for decent health care and a brave exposing of an inner life, *The Soul of Care* gives language for what we all crave – effective, generous health care that nourishes those who give and those who receive until they recognize their oneness' Rita Charon, Columbia Narrative Medicine

'A rich account of care as presence, immediacy and attention that should matter to our medical system. But above all it is a love story – of great pain, but also of joy. It is about what really matters in our lives' T. M. Luhrmann, author of *Of Two Minds: An Anthropologist Looks at American Psychiatry*

'Arthur Kleinman's very human story is an inspiration for all of us' Lee Goldman, Dean of Columbia University School of Medicine

'What was at stake for Arthur in his caring for Joan was nothing short of his humanity. Read this book and prepare to be both humbled and inspired' Jim Yong Kim, Former President of the World Bank

'One of our nation's most humane doctors and profound thinkers has insightful, moving, and novel things to say about our capacity to give and get care. Powerful, intimate, poignant, and helpful' Nicholas A. Christakis, author of *Blueprint: The Evolutionary Origins of a Good Society*

'A love story for the ages, a moral treatise, and a devastating critique of the absence of care in modern institutions and relationships' Tahmima Anam, author of *The Bones of Grace*

ABOUT THE AUTHOR

Arthur Kleinman is one of the most renowned and influential experts on psychiatry, global health and cultural issues in medicine. He is currently a professor of psychiatry and of medical anthropology at Harvard Medical School and Esther and Sidney Rabb Professor of Anthropology. Having spent decades doing field research in China and Taiwan, he is also a leading expert on East Asia. He is the author of *The Illness Narratives: Suffering, Healing and the Human Condition*, now widely used in medical schools.

ARTHUR KLEINMAN

The Soul of Care

The Moral Education of a Doctor

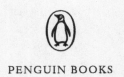

PENGUIN BOOKS

PENGUIN BOOKS

UK | USA | Canada | Ireland | Australia
India | New Zealand | South Africa

Penguin Books is part of the Penguin Random House group of companies
whose addresses can be found at global.penguinrandomhouse.com

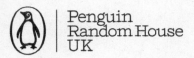

First published in the United States of America by Viking 2019
First published in Great Britain by Penguin Books 2020
001

Copyright © Arthur Kleinman, 2019

Printed in Great Britain by Clays Ltd, Elcograf S.p.A.

A CIP catalogue record for this book is available from the British Library

ISBN: 978-0-141-99241-9

www.greenpenguin.co.uk

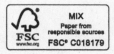

Penguin Random House is committed to a
sustainable future for our business, our readers
and our planet. This book is made from Forest
Stewardship Council® certified paper.

Information contained in this book accurately conveys the spirit of my work as a physician, an anthropologist, and a family caregiver. With the exception of autobiographical details, family members, and primary care physicians and hospitals who took care of Joan Kleinman, all names and identifying details in the case histories have been changed. This is meant to ensure confidentiality and to protect the anonymity of the individuals, families, and institutions involved. When I have made such changes, I have drawn on information from other patients, research subjects, and physicians facing similar problems to make the alteration valid in the light of the experiences of people I have treated, studied, and worked with.

The Soul *of* Care

Prologue

G et out! Get out!"
My wife, Joan, is screaming, and hitting out wildly at the stranger in her bed. She is greatly agitated and frightened. "Get away from here. Get out!"

But the man she perceives as a stranger is me, her husband of more than forty years. Joan has just woken up from a midday nap. It is summer 2009 in Cambridge, Massachusetts. We are in the bedroom of the home we have lived in for twenty-seven years.

I try to keep my voice calm and hide the panic rising inside me. "I'm your husband, Arthur. Don't be so upset, I'm here with you!"

"You are not! You are not Arthur! You are an impostor! Get out! Now!" she yells, shaking and intensely alert, like a trapped animal.

I try in all the ways I can think of to calm her and to prove to her that I am indeed her husband, but she insists, denying who I am, growing more and more adamant, more and more upset. I begin to wonder if this is real or if I have woken up in a nightmare. Joan feels only terror, caught in the grip of a delusion that frightens her to the core. This has happened once before, in a hotel in Amsterdam the previous year, but still I feel totally unprepared to deal with her delirium.

Joan is almost blind and suffers dementia as a result of an atypical kind of early-onset Alzheimer's disease. This excruciating episode is a classic manifestation of Capgras syndrome, a delusional state that occurs sometimes in people suffering neurodegenerative disorders. The affected person systematically misperceives those close to her and even the physical space she is occupying as unreal and fake. As in Joan's case, it most often is episodic, short-lived, and readily forgotten, but for those close to the sufferer, it can be world-shattering—as if a bond that has taken decades to forge can be broken in an instant.

I'm a trained psychiatrist. I should have the tools to deal with this. But right now, in this moment, I am a shocked and devastated husband. This episode, like the first, lasts a few terrible hours. During that time, I have to retreat to another part of our house, and wait until it burns itself out and she has returned to a calm state. I am also, however, a caregiver—Joan's primary caregiver. Several times I try to engage her in normal conversation, but she rejects me. Finally, I make believe I am someone else, there to help her.

"Well, get rid of this impostor and find my real husband," she implores.

Afterward she made light of it. The very next day, she denied that it had happened at all. Up to this point, I had been caring for Joan for eight years. I had helped bathe, dress, and guide her. I also had to help her with eating and increasingly with interpreting the world for her. I was an ordinary family carer, one of more than fifty million in the United States at any time. But I have also

THE SOUL OF CARE

devoted my career as a physician and medical anthropologist to professional care and studying caregiving. I have objective expertise in this subject, and at the same time, I am immersed in it as an ordinary participant, learning every day as I go.

From each of these experiences, but particularly from the terrible decade I spent as a family carer, I gained a deeper understanding of caregiving. I found that care is a human development process. Often in our society, boys are raised to be careless, girls to be careful. It takes a long time for adolescent and young men to learn to care about others and then become caring, and at last give care. While the social pressure and cultural expectations of women to be carers is much greater, it doesn't mean care is natural or easier for them. Women develop as carers too. Care is centered in relationships. Caregiving and receiving is a gift-sharing process in which we give and receive attention, affirmation, practical assistance, emotional support, moral solidarity, and abiding meaning that is complicated and incomplete. Care is action, practice, performance. Often it is *reaction*. A constant reaction to the needs of others and ourselves under different conditions and in different contexts. Care is accompanying someone through their experiences of alarm and injury. It is assisting, protecting, thinking ahead to prevent further difficulty.

Care is also about the vital *presence*—the liveliness and fullness of being—of both the caregiver and the care recipient. Acts of caring call that presence out from within us. Care does not end with death but involves actively caring for memories. I learned that caregiving entails moments of terror and panic, of self-doubt and hopelessness—but also moments of deep human connection, of honesty and revelation, of purpose and gratification.

I also learned how far the domain of caregiving extends beyond the boundaries of medicine. Caregiving is perhaps the most ubiquitous activity of human beings, and it can be the most demanding, at times discouraging, one. It is also the existential activity through which we most fully realize our humanity. In the humblest moments of caring—mopping a sweaty brow, changing a soiled sheet, reassuring an agitated person, kissing the cheek of a loved one at the end of life—we may embody the finest versions of ourselves. It can offer redemption to the caregiver and the person to whom he is giving care. Care can offer wisdom for the art of living.

Caregiving is hard, sometimes tedious, unglamorous work, but it resonates with emotional, moral, and even religious significance. Understanding the meanings that arise from the practical work of care may help us to meet the challenges of sustaining it, and of enduring its many trials, and also may strengthen us to face the other tests that life brings. Those challenges are increasing. I believe we are living through a dangerous time when high-quality care is seriously threatened among families, in the health professions, in our hospitals and aged care homes, and in our society at large. Amid the hardness, hate, violence, and cynicism that fuel politics today, an anti-caring ethos prevails, and undermined by funding that scarcely touches the need, care can be wrongly portrayed as softness and sentimentality. It is neither. Care is the human glue that holds together families, communities, and societies. Care offers an alternative story of how we live and who we are. But it is being silenced and diminished in value, in the United States and around the world, sacrificed on the altar of economy and efficiency, demanding more and more of families and health care professionals with fewer and fewer resources, and threatening to displace meaning in health care. The moral language of human experience, of people's suffering and healing—

the bedrock of our common existence—is being stifled, and at worst will be lost.

We must be prepared to ask uncomfortable questions of ourselves, to challenge the assumptions of our institutions and the premises of the "health care debate." It is a time to act. This volume is my testament about caregiving and why it matters most.

One

Not much in my youth signaled a future of caregiving.

I never knew my biological father, Nathan Spier. Even as I write his name, I am unable to conjure a face or even a shadow. My mother, Marcia, ran away from him and from a marriage she couldn't tolerate, taking me with her, when I was one. I didn't know his full name or anything else about him until I was in my twenties, and even then, the subject remained radioactive enough in my family that I made no serious effort to find him. The mystery of my origins would haunt much of my young life. My own mother was unable to talk to me about my biological father and his family until she was in her sixties, and even then, she insisted that I should never meet him. A real estate developer, called the King of Bensonhurst as I later learned, he and his family had been involved in a scandal concerning illegal influence on the courts that resulted in the suicide of a judge. And to this day, that is all I permitted myself to know.

I grew up in a well-to-do Jewish family, in an economically and culturally mixed Brooklyn neighborhood. Our household, at least initially, consisted of my mother, my maternal grandparents, and me. My mother was a vivacious redhead (dyed) who loved the high life filled with nights out on the town, which she balanced with volunteer work in hospitals and for Jewish advocacy groups. She had the means to hire nurses and maids to look after me and, later, my brother. When she realized that I had played hooky from Hebrew school for several weeks, she assured me that I would indeed learn enough Hebrew to achieve my bar mitzvah, because she would not be denied the privilege of throwing a big party, as was expected in her circle. She made it clear throughout my childhood that I was to become a physician or a professor, or some other high-status professional whose intellectual achievements would add a patina of class and respectability to the family's financial success.

My mother was also high-strung and volatile. I never doubted her love, but at the same time, I found her emotionally untrustworthy. When my half brother came along, I never felt sure if her concern for me was as great as her worry about him. I sensed that she and the rest of the family saw me as more self-sufficient and able to look after myself. My stepfather would prove to be almost as much of a party animal as my mother, and their friendship networks included all kinds of colorful and sometimes slightly shady characters.

My mother was one of four daughters, but her father's clear favorite. It was for this reason that we lived with my grandparents. My grandfather, a proudly secular Jew of Russian background, had built a prosperous soap company and amassed real estate holdings. His business prospered in the 1930s and early '40s but went into precipitous decline in the postwar years.

My grandfather was, I imagine, typical for his times, but would seem totally out of place in the second decade of the twenty-first century. He was formal, distant, and authoritarian. He didn't express his love in words but in deeds, protecting and often defending me when neighbors and shopkeepers objected to my delinquent behavior. I remember one Saturday morning, when the Lubavitcher Rebbe, Menachem Mendel Schneerson, a monumental figure in the Hasidic Jewish community who had recently moved next door, took away the basketball I was dribbling and told me not to play on the Sabbath. It was my grandfather who retrieved my basketball from the Rebbe and admonished me to play with it outside *every* Saturday from then on. He was at the very center of the family—a loving *paterfamilias*—and he carried as an almost sacred duty the responsibility for our financial and social security. I admired my grandfather, and always felt secure under his protective wing but never felt emotionally close to him.

In contrast to my high-living mother, my grandmother was old-world, a poorly educated, superstitious, and increasingly paranoid matriarch who never left the house and who occasionally whispered to me that I came from an even richer family. Her mysterious mutterings only further confused and disturbed me, since she would stubbornly refuse to elaborate, no matter how hard I questioned her.

These older generations saw me as a willful, headstrong little boy, naturally resistant to authority. In the family's folklore, these traits were forged at birth, when I emerged from the birth canal with the umbilical cord wrapped tightly around my neck, blue and struggling to breathe. In their eyes, I was born a fighter, and it's fair to say that I did little to dissuade them from that notion as I grew up.

In 1943, when I was two years old, my mother absconded with me to Miami, so as to thwart my biological father, who was trying to use legal means to compel our return. (Apparently, Florida did not recognize New York State's marriage laws then.) For a while we lived across from a hostel for army and navy officers, several of whom took an interest in my mother. I remember asking each one plaintively but with hope, "Are you my father?" Perhaps this sense of loss and longing contributed more to my aggressive will-fulness than any birth trauma I might have experienced. At any rate, my behavior got bad enough that my frustrated kindergarten teacher insisted my mother remove me from the classroom. "He only does things his own way," she complained.

My mother met the man who would become my stepfather during that brief sojourn in Florida. Peter Kleinman had played professional basketball and was a minor celebrity in his day. He was good-looking, friendly and charming, and admired by many. I admired him, too, when I was young. As I grew older, though, I could see that my grandfather regarded him as a failure in busi-ness and in his law practice, and with good reason. I think even my mother, who loved her new husband, came to share this view. I could feel my stepfather's love and concern for me—he was the man I saw as my dad—but I understood and accepted that he loved my brother, his natural son, more. Peter Kleinman would adopt me when I was twelve, changing my name from Arthur Spier (pronounced "Spear") to Arthur Kleinman, so that it felt as if I was starting out anew.

In the decade after my grandfather's death in 1958, during which time my stepfather stopped working, he and my mother together spent her entire inheritance. I didn't feel the loss of the family's financial security as deeply as the resentment, embar-rassment, and maybe even shame over the irresponsibility of my parents, who had put the family—meaning my brother and me—second. This was quite the opposite of the example set by my grandfather.

My kindergarten teacher wasn't completely wrong about me. I remember an episode from around that same time, when I angrily informed my mother I was running away from home. When my mother opened the door I had so dramatically slammed on the way out, she found me sitting on the steps. I couldn't go any further, I explained, because I was not allowed to cross the street on my own! Clearly, there was something in my nature, even at this early time, which acted as a natural brake on my impulsiveness. I could be difficult, but I knew there were rules and directives that needed to be followed. And I was not so foolhardy as to do something that would cause me to injure myself. This fundamental awareness would keep me out of trouble time and again during my childhood, or at least it helped keep that trouble to a mostly manageable level.

Back in Brooklyn, I attended a public school four blocks from our house. Our Crown Heights neighborhood was a mainly Jewish enclave surrounded by Irish and Italian communities, where apartment blocks thrust their dark brick facades from between brighter rows of sturdy single-family houses. In the street, we boys played stickball or punchball, bought vanilla or chocolate cones from the ice cream truck, shot marbles, flipped coins, watched the girls play hopscotch, experimented with cigarettes, and fought with one another to see who was the toughest. Nobody bothered to hide their racism or anti-Semitism in the 1940s and early '50s, and I got into many fights on the streets outside our little enclave on account of being Jewish and unwilling, to a point anyway, to back down. But there must have been more than this at stake for me because I fought with Jewish boys too.

My life on the street from 1944 to 1953 contrasted sharply with the cushy existence at home, where we had a cook and a housekeeper and I never had so much as a chore to do. I was given to understand that I would always be financially secure and that the family would always take care of me—not exactly the best message to encourage my sense of responsibility and stewardship.

I treated myself from childhood on with a carelessness that was surely compounded by my mother's distraction with a new marriage that had produced a new child. I neglected my health, as did most kids then, I suppose, and have suffered the consequences ever since, with dental problems, asthma, melanoma, and other ailments.

My neighborhood friends came from hardworking ethnic families, and most were not well off like mine. I spent my childhood with these tough working-class kids, instinctively understanding that the best way to survive the bullies and the street fighters was to become one of them. I learned to take care of myself, teasing, hassling, and abusing other kids just for the sport of it. I was becoming not just tough, but hard.

And yet that same instinct that kept me from crossing the street when I wanted to run away from home must have also tempered the worst of my behavior toward others. It was partly a nascent awareness of the need for self-protective boundaries, but also an awakening sense of the emotional and moral responsibilities of relationships. Around age ten or eleven, when girls started to come into focus, I developed a childhood crush on one in particular. But the conventions of courtship entirely escaped me. I think I must have believed that I had the right to help myself to whatever captured my fancy. At the end of the school day as we all left to walk home, I asked her if I could carry her books. It never occurred to me that I might be rebuffed, and when she said "No!" I impulsively grabbed the books and ran away. It took only a few moments to recognize I had done something shameful and for a hopeful suitor terminally unhelpful, so I returned her books with a burning feeling in my face and chest.

At the same age, an older boy in the playground tried to wrench my brand-new basketball from my hands. When I refused to let go, he banged my head repeatedly against the steel pole that supported the hoop. My head was bleeding, but I refused to cry in front of him or the other kids who had gathered around, or beg for the ball back. I ran home believing my dignity was still intact but bearing the wounds of battle. I wasn't angry about the injustice done to me; I was just burning for revenge. I would show I would not be trifled with or cowed. I would strike back. I had watched and learned. But all I had really learned is what every bully knows: you pick fights with those you can defeat and humiliate.

I came to the cynical understanding that beneath its orderly and proper exterior, it is a violent world without justice or goodness. I learned another brutal lesson, also not compatible with caregiving, in a fight with another aggressive boy who lived on the block. Following a minute of grappling and hitting, I locked my arms around his head and squeezed as hard as I could. He started to cry and begged me to stop. So I released my hold, only to have him crush my neck with a hammerlock that was so tight I couldn't breathe. I gave up, and he celebrated his victory by laughing at me. It would take me a long time to unlearn the lesson this particular beating taught me: to resist empathizing with my enemies, to take no pity, no mercy.

Every now and then, though, the light found its way through a crack in my armor. One summer when I was eleven or twelve, I had gone to a summer camp in upstate New York, where I joined with the other more rugged campers in making fun of a small, bespectacled boy who avoided sports and always carried a book around. But his surprising response to our teasing—arguing that he was becoming serious about intellectual matters—was so passionate, so mature, and yet carried lightly with a self-deprecating humor that I felt a respect and even admiration for him. This boy was also caring. When I got hit in the head with a softball pitch, he ran over to see if I was all right. I knew I liked him and what he stood for, which was so very different from the rest of my experience. I couldn't recall having felt that way before, except for the tough kids whose coarse behavior I emulated. I remember wondering if there might be a way to be like him and also still be myself. This was one of the first times in my life that I actually began to see that there was a part of me that wasn't being cultivated at all, and perhaps was even being stifled by my hard shell.

Yet even on those tough streets occasionally there was evidence that friends had your back, at least when you were threatened by *"outsiders,"* such as kids from other neighborhoods, older kids who belonged to rival gangs, or the police. I remember a time when everybody knew about a big gang fight among high schoolers that was to take place in a park near my school. I was very excited and planned to go. Two of my friends prevented me from going, insisting that if I got involved, even as an observer, I was likely to get into more serious trouble. At a nearby movie theater for a Saturday matinee, a fight started several rows behind where I was sitting with friends. I started out of my seat to take a closer look at the action, but one of my classmates abruptly pulled me back by the collar of my jacket, saying, "Come on, they have knives. We are getting out of here!" Could we call these school chums and street friends a social network that functioned as a caring circle? If I had used words like these with them I doubtless would have been laughed at and ridiculed. But there was a kind of incipient care among us that held fast despite the otherwise brutal atmosphere of carelessness and violence. We shared a local world, and knew it, and we were learning how to care for one another.

It was at this time, however, that it suddenly became clear that the street persona I had developed had not gone unnoticed in our little corner of Brooklyn. The cops on the beat brought me to the boxing program in the Police Athletic League as a way of redirecting my aggression. And more troublingly, a local man singled me out as a kid with potential. He came up to me on the sidewalk one day and playfully mussed my hair while telling me that he had his eye on me. Shortly after, I spied a newspaper photo of him in police custody, with a headline identifying him as a leading Mafia enforcer. Whether it was that single event or the larger constellation of concerns about our neighborhood, my associates, and my waywardness, my grandfather and my parents concluded that it was time to get me out of that world. They decided to leave Brooklyn and move the family to the suburbs on Long Island.

In my new school, I channeled my overbearing drive into academic work. This was a fiercely competitive setting, but now the competition was for educational success and recognition. Like me, my fellow students were on the way up, climbing aggressively and not much given to empathy or real friendships. The tough boys of Brooklyn were replaced by the ambitious boys—and girls—of our new neighborhood. And I was to find that the rules of engagement were very different. I actually got into a scuffle on my first day at the new school, taking down a couple of bullies who confronted me and warned me about showing off with my smart answers in the classroom. I was shocked when my triumph horrified the other kids, rather than eliciting their respect.

These developments came together with several others to push my life in a new direction. First, I became an avid reader and—guided by several teachers and others who took a major interest in me, including a diminutive older woman who invited me to a reading by poets at her Greenwich Village apartment—I educated myself in history and literature. I was especially drawn to personal narratives: biographies, autobiographies, memoirs, journals. In each of these I searched for the ways the context affected real lives, and historical contingencies altered genetic ones. This was my precocious and dizzying exposure to Dostoevsky's "fire in the minds of men" and its local misadventures—revolutions intensifying social suffering, destroyed by corruption and bad faith, and the ironies and failures that are constant in human experience and that unbend the arc of justice and further break broken men. It was too much wisdom too early, yet it had its effect. I was furnishing the soul of a youngster who would come to the understanding that what was missing in the world was care for ordinary people. Alan Paton's *Cry, the Beloved Country*, Graham Greene's *The Power and the Glory* and *The Heart of the Matter*, George Orwell's *Down and Out in Paris and London*, *The Road to Wigan Pier*, *Homage to Catalonia*, and *Animal Farm*, and other works became more real to me than my historical times—the dull, conformist, and predictable 1950s. I didn't understand how rare it would become to have a whole weekend—because there was no TV, no social media—to get wrapped up in a novel or a travel story or social history.

And second, I developed a passionate and abiding interest in the stories of those around me: the real people in my life. This surely was abetted by my confusion about my own story. Who was I anyway? Were the incomplete fragments of stories I was picking up from my grandmother and my mother true or not? Where did they lead? And since I was prohibited from crossing over to the other side of my ancestry, did it really matter if I couldn't figure it out? The stultifying 1950s had also seen the rising influence of existentialism, and I had developed in my teens the core doubt that any of this history really mattered. If the world was absurd, wasn't my biography yet one more instance of just how absurd it could be? Later I would see this as the central point of *Man's Search for Meaning*, the seminal book by the psychiatrist, neurologist, and Holocaust survivor Viktor Frankl: we can't control what has happened to us, yet we can control how we think about it, and so make it meaningful in our lives.

There was also my dawning recognition in the 1950s that even though we were still wealthy, history was conspiring to reduce that wealth in a macroeconomic way that we could not control. The new suburbia destroyed the value of my grandfather's investment in inner cities. Liquid soap came to replace hard soap in public toilets, undermining the family's soap business. The square block on the east side of midtown Manhattan that my grandfather had purchased as a safety net was taken away by Tammany Hall politicians under eminent domain. At the time, these historical contingencies were invisible, covered over with the uncertain anxieties of the lived experience of our days, camouflaged by the one-damn-thing-after-another ordinariness of our lives.

I learned to be an intense listener, a sharp observer of people's struggles to make sense of their worlds and themselves. I didn't realize it at the time, but I suppose I had intuitively begun to train myself in the rudiments of psychiatry. And I was a natural ethnographer, even though I had never at the time heard this word. My deep curiosity about how people lived their lives and turned their experiences into particular meanings about what was at stake for them transformed me from a self-conscious, immature teenager worried about his pimples and moles into a questioning, informed, experience-oriented student of human conditions. As I listened and people talked, I learned to hear not only their words but also their human tone.

So the small bohemian middle-aged woman, the intellectual who invited me to her studio apartment in Greenwich Village to hear poets of the Beat Generation, confided in me that she was an alcoholic and had experimented with all the drugs she could find because she had failed to escape to Europe and find her artistic destiny, making her feel she had "murdered her life." I listened; her words inscribed themselves in me, but how could I understand their sad meaning?

Or when our maid Hatty, the tall, unflappable African American woman who had raised me from age four, told me when I was fifteen that every day she had spent with me represented a day she had failed to spend with her own son and daughter. That was the first and only time she didn't laugh when she picked up after me, but broke down in angry tears. And although I truly believed I had always loved her, it was the first time I had heard the tone of her pain and saw through the cruel fiction of her being "a member of the family."

Then there was my neighbor: an attractive young married woman whose husband had suffered a heart attack and was now confined to a wheelchair. She asked me to listen to her as she gave vent to her frustration, her sadness, and his hopelessness. She didn't know how they would survive this sudden devastating trauma. Why did she tell me, a sixteen-year-old, these awful truths? Maybe she could only have told someone like me, who had nothing to offer except witnessing her miserable condition, because all I could do was reflect back her fear and feel her desperation. From the vantage of six decades on, it would seem she had recognized something responsive in me that needed to be aware of the cost of caregiving for another. Notably, no one my own age acted this way with me; only older people did, and almost always they were women.

These women, among others, were in retrospect training me as an adolescent to listen, witness, and safely share my presence with them. I was awakening to the understanding that their personal problems were social ills that were shared with others in my world and grew out of the history and culture in which they lived, as much as from the particular lives they led. I was being brought into a different emotional sensibility and new kinds of moral relationships, ones where caring mattered and the act of recognizing or creating meaning was a way of giving and receiving love.

Over the years, the confining, parochial world of the neighborhood, my family, their business enterprises, and their expectations of me became oppressive. I could no longer abide the narrow, self-interested, pragmatic talk about making money (not something I had ever had to try to accomplish, of course) and the lack of engagement with substantive ideas and moral questions. Sure, there was a genuine concern with the plight of Jews in the world, but even that struck me as a tribal, exclusive interest that ignored social justice for other groups, including the weak and vulnerable in our own city.

As soon as I could, I escaped that place, first to Tufts University in New England and then to the West Coast and Stanford for college and later medical school. I was in college and professional school at an extraordinary time: The civil rights, antiwar, and feminist movements were growing rapidly, upending values long taken for granted, and introducing the idea that the society and individuals in it (like me) needed to undergo radical change. My fellow students were going off to organize African American voters in the South, campaign against the Vietnam War, protest patriarchy and male chauvinism, and invent original forms of aesthetic and emotional expression. Later on, I would realize that it was the United States—not China, where the phrase was coined—that experienced a genuine "cultural revolution." Everything seemed possible, not least personal transformation.

As a fledgling intellectual, I discovered Albert Camus, and felt he was a moral icon of the responsibility to engage the great issue of one's time. I read the literature of the European Left, who were still wrestling with the aftermath of fascism and collaboration and were searching for new forms of solidarity with, and support of, the poor and the marginal. I was taught by Malcolm Cowley—novelist and literary critic who had chronicled the "lost generation" of American writers after World War I in Europe—who insisted that Hemingway, Fitzgerald, and others had to be understood as born into a time they could not master but that had broken and redeemed them. I wrote the words in my notebook, but I was not ready for their wisdom.

The literature I valued mirrored my growing awareness that I would someday pivot like Shakespeare's Prince Hal from the young wastrel in *Henry IV* to the victorious warrior king in *Henry V*. Just like him I would turn away from my troubling past but draw on it to create a more successful future. So it was no surprise that Joseph Conrad's *Lord Jim* and *Victory* were among my favorites. Each presented a hero who early in his life had failed to muster the courage and responsibility needed to face a crisis in his local world and had run away to a foreign place where he was unknown and could remake his life entirely. Having succeeded in this new world, he eventually had to face once again a crisis that required him to stand up to a dangerous evil threatening him and those he had come to love. The romanticism of this life trajectory never bothered me. Instead, I took the message to mean that I, too, could redeem a wanton and thoughtless childhood, and use what had strengthened me physically and psychologically in a totally different way that might do good in the world.

Looking back, I sense I had an inkling of what that new life would be. It was Sinclair Lewis's *Arrowsmith* and Axel Munthe's *The Story of San Michele*, tales of young doctors (one even a psychiatrist) finding meaning in their lives through work and love.

Later, other important books would continue this central interest in the transformation of young lives and their moral development, especially Thomas Mann's *Buddenbrooks* and *The Magic Mountain*.

And at the same time, I marveled at the majestic beauty of California's Big Sur, and felt personally liberated enough to become aware that I had a longing to be loved and an urgent need to love in return. I never found love among the mist-covered and rock-strewn beaches, the turquoise ocean, the huge redwoods, but I did encounter other seekers—students who like me confused the search for the pleasures of romance with moral and spiritual quests. I recognized the confusion underlying the adventures of many of my peers, but I remained blind to the futility in my own quest. I was also ready for a new direction, something that could unite my intellectual aspirations with the practical orientation of the medical training I was preparing to pursue. I was searching for what would come to matter most in my life. It would prove to be a complicated but transformative journey.

Romance became a constant preoccupation. Since my teenage years, I had resisted the building pressure to date the Jewish girls from moneyed backgrounds to whom I was repeatedly introduced. One blind date arranged by my mother's friends was with the daughter of a major company CEO who lived in a penthouse on Fifth Avenue and whose father explained to me the purchase price and current value of an original Picasso painting, the only thing in his living room that he seemed to even notice. I felt he was appraising me in the same way. I wanted to date whatever girl I wanted. Here my powerful inner need to be loved merged with a rising sense that beautiful, educated, and sophisticated Protestant women were the ones who could do that and at the same time remove me from a cloying upper-middle-class ethnic ghetto.

Having relocated myself, both physically and spiritually, and having become newly familiar with Marxist teachings, I started to think about the world in a different way. In solidarity with the workingman—or so I thought—I took a summer job in the New York City sewer system. The sewers were a dank and dark netherworld under the streets, the workplace of an army of engineers and laborers, unseen and unappreciated by those aboveground. And it was a forbidding place. My boss was an example of all that was wrong with society, I thought. Bigoted, untrustworthy, and corrupt, he berated my fellow workers and encouraged bad behavior among them, like pilfering, shirking duties, and falsely claiming overtime.

Bill Burt, a large, white-haired Irishman who reminded me of Robert Louis Stevenson's description of Long John Silver—"boisterous and piratical"—mentored me in how to adapt to the sewers and to our appalling boss. At the same time, he taught me about life on a grander scale. Despite the limits of a dreadful job that he couldn't wait to escape from through early retirement, it seemed to me he was a kind of secular saint, helping others and standing up for the weakest of them. He protected me and held me to the standards that made me a competent worker. A good man and the first person with whom I fully shared my fears and aspirations, Bill was also the first person I felt I could trust emotionally to offer me the wisdom and care of an older man for a younger apprentice.

The school year at Stanford that followed my summer in the sewer was my first year of medical school, and I found I couldn't abide the tedious study of basic science that the training required. Indulging myself in righteous indignation, I wrote Bill a rambling, sentimental letter, explaining that I was thinking of dropping out to become a blue-collar worker like him, and also try my hand at writing. He wrote me back, in vernacular almost entirely devoid of punctuation and grammar, asking me if I wanted "to do donkey labor like me the rest of your life?" He admonished me not to lose my chance in life, ending, "Kid, if you give up becoming a doctor, I'll come there and break your legs!" The bracing response had the immediate salutary effect of keeping me focused on my path, but the care this father figure expressed for me held a lesson that would only come clear to me years down the road.

During those early years in medical school, two experiences abroad awakened me to a subject that I would pursue throughout my career, the suffering that so many societies endure and its aftermath for vulnerable individuals. I took a trip to Germany in 1963, happily traveling with fellow students and not thinking much beyond my own self-absorbed concerns, when I arrived in Alsace in France, and checked in at a small hotel in a tiny village. Wandering along the canals outside the village, I was forced by a passing rainstorm to run to a copse of trees and ended up stepping into a hidden cemetery. There I found a small monument to a multigenerational family, all of whose members had the same wartime date of death. When I got back I asked the hotel's receptionist in German—I should have used French but I didn't possess it then—about this grim oddity. She shouted at me that it was my people, the Germans, who had killed this family. This was at a time when there was little attention paid to the Holocaust in the United States, and I had hardly thought or talked about being a Jew in Germany, only eighteen years after the war's end. Thus, my first encounter with the Shoah was, in her eyes at least, as a perpetrator. This troubling experience broke through my self-absorption. It was the first time I truly felt the overwhelming dangers of the world from which my privileged life had protected me, and the responsibility we have to honor history and bear witness to human suffering.

The second experience grew from this one. Horrified by my willful ignorance and the possibility that I could be taken for one of the guilty, I went directly to Israel that summer to confront my Jewish identity. There I became the object of an intense recruitment effort by the charismatic leader of a kibbutz. He entreated me to join the other young Jews from around the world who were building a future in the desert. I declined. In reacting to his enthusiastic presentation of Zionism, I came to realize that I was more at home in the plural, diverse world of the Diaspora and felt uncomfortable with ethnic, national, and religious exclusivity. Yet I still didn't recognize at the time that the trajectory of my own life was slowly bending in a direction that likely would have surprised, if not astounded, my early teachers and friends, including the likes of Bill Burt and certainly that Mafia recruiter.

These early experiences have become touchstones for interpreting the way my life and work have unfolded. In the years that followed I became a physician, a husband, a father, a writer, and a teacher. Perhaps because of my psychiatric training and clinical experience, I still seek meaning in the formative experiences of childhood and youth, not least my own. I can look back on those years and recognize that I entered early adulthood having not yet learned to care for myself and for others, that I was careless and simply expected to be cared for, that I had only partially reformed myself, and that even though I read and wrote about care, I had not yet practiced caregiving, not in the family, not even in the medical profession.

Two

Surely, it had to have been more than my family's expectations that steered me toward medicine. It wasn't as if we had a tradition of physicians in the family or even had doctors in our social circles. But the one doctor who did figure in my early life made a great impression on me.

Dr. Frederick Ben was a stern but gentle general practitioner who treated my frequent childhood and adolescent chest infections, often in my own home. Dr. Ben looked every inch the European doctor, pleasantly plump, with close-cropped hair, a neatly trimmed beard, bushy eyebrows, and rimless eyeglasses framing his kind but piercing eyes. His heavy tweed blazer and gray flannel pants were always redolent with the aroma of pipe tobacco. He spoke in thickly accented English, with the rather formal cadences of his native German, occasionally signaling a shift from dispassionate medical commentary to more intimate words of personal wisdom by passing his hand across his face and shaking his head. I don't remember Dr. Ben smiling that often, but I do remember the mixture of concern, careful attention, and earnest encouragement in his expression as he percussed my chest and listened intently to my lungs through his stethoscope.

A few times, Dr. Ben and his wife invited me to take tea and cake with them in the living room of the house where he lived, in which he also had his office and examining rooms. On these occasions, he would share his experiences with me, although only rarely did he allude to the anti-Semitism he and his family must have faced before emigrating from Nazi Germany. Instead, he regaled me with clinical accounts of memorable cases, spinning them like medical detective stories. One theme that seemed to underlie many of these stories was the woeful absence of effective treatments. After all, even as recently as the mid-1950s, there weren't many truly reliable medical treatments for serious diseases. Penicillin had only just become widespread in medical practice. Dr. Ben himself used to hand out "red" and "blue" pills to almost all of his adolescent patients. He did this so often and so readily, without ever explaining what the pills were, that my brother and I suspected they were just placebos.

As I grew into my mid-teens, Dr. Ben started subtly recruiting me for a career in medicine. He saw medicine, first and foremost, as a moral calling. It was about doing good for people who needed help. The technical details mattered greatly, but Dr. Ben believed in the doctor-patient relationship as the vital core of medical practice. He once told me that if a doctor earned the complete trust of a patient, the doctor could talk the patient out of an acute attack of asthma, reduce the pain of gouty arthritis, even mobilize a demoralized cancer patient into action. He attributed such marvels to the charismatic presence of the physician and the ability to draw vitality and healing power out of the patient's inner self.

Dr. Ben impressed on me the importance of the home visits he made. He would explain that these house calls enabled him to observe the patient's and family's intimate domestic space. He was careful not to exaggerate the significance of either the home visits or the role of the doctor-patient relationship in the healing process, but I understood that above all, he valued the humanness inherent in these practices. His idealistic view of medicine, or at least its potential, had a strong influence on me. It resonated with my parents' overly romantic notion that the practice of medicine differed from business, law, or engineering because it functioned primarily to help people and to improve the world. Over time, I internalized these values, so that when I began studying medicine myself, my expectations for clinical work were high.

My calling to care started to come into focus when I got to work directly with patients. One of the first I encountered was a seven-year-old girl in a rehabilitation unit. She was covered in horrific burns over much of her body. In my book *The Illness Narratives* I recounted how each day, she endured excruciating debridement, a treatment in which she was put into a whirlpool bath so that the burned tissue could be painstakingly removed from her wounds. It was a wrenching ordeal, both for her and for the medical team, which included me at the very bottom of the clinical hierarchy. Screaming with pain and fear of more pain, she fought the doctors and nurses, begging them not to hurt her anymore. My job as a medical student was to hold her unburned hand—to calm her so that the surgical resident could continue to debride her wounds. Those extensive patches of burned flesh bled, turning the water in the whirlpool first pink, then a deep, garish crimson.

This sweet, frail little girl, her face disfigured and her body just one big scar, would cry out in terror and pain, wailing that pained me to hear: "It hurts. It hurts so bad. Help me! Help me! Please help me make them stop! Don't touch me!" I struggled to distract this little patient's attention away from this daily suffering. I asked her about her family and home life, her experiences at school, her friends or hobbies, anything I could think of that might help this hypervigilant girl escape the agony mentally, so that the surgeon and the nurse could do their work. I myself could hardly bear the visceral experience of her torment: the screams, the burned skin, the bloody water, her daily battle with the nurses over the care of her wounds.

Desperate to make her feel better and assist the staff, I felt helpless and inept. Then one day I broke through, almost by accident: I asked her to explain to me how she could tolerate the situation she was in, each and every day. For the first time, she stopped screaming and spoke directly to me. She stopped fighting the surgeon and the nurses. But now, having established a real connection, she spoke in a calmer though still anguished voice. "Don't let go! Stay here!" And then, squeezing my hand, she went on to tell me about her pain: the sharp sting of the whirlpool, the misery of the ointments and bandages, the comfort she felt in the bed that made her desperate to stay there, even when she knew she couldn't. Looking at her, listening to her, broke my heart. She drew out of me an overwhelming desire to comfort her, but not with trite words of hope. No, what she wanted from me was intense listening, and for me to speak to her with the same directness with which she so courageously spoke to me. Doubtless, I didn't always get it right, but I endured because she endured. I was with her in that hell that no child should ever have to endure.

From that day forward, we established a kind of trust. Each day, she held my hand and opened up to me about what she felt as she again went through the harrowing surgical ritual. During my time on this clinical unit, I saw that I had a positive effect on this little burned patient's response to her care, but her impact on me was so much greater. I learned from her a clinical truth that has well served both me and the patients I have met: Even when patients are in crisis—perhaps especially when they are in crisis—you can talk with them about what matters most in their lives, as revealed in their response to illness and treatment. It isn't easy, but you can build a relationship of emotional and moral resonance that brings both the doctor and the patient (and often the family as well) to the heart of care.

Patients like this gave me moments of awakening during my medical education, and these moments set free the passions that would become my lifework. Although they had little to do with my classes and textbooks, they transformed me and opened my eyes to why care went beyond simple diagnosis and treatment. Care was equally about sharing and witnessing the lived experience of pain and suffering, the victories and disappointments that comprise the flow of illness and treatment.

An elderly white-haired woman, her beauty still apparent in her fine features, came into the Stanford Hospital clinic. I remember how she turned red with shame as she revealed to me that she had acquired syphilis during World War I from a sexual encounter with a soldier who had recently returned from the battlefield in France. The only treatment available in the days before penicillin was Salvarsan, an arsenic compound that had had terrible side effects on her body. The liver damage she suffered had turned her skin yellow. With her discolored skin, her fear that the disease would affect her brain, and because she mistakenly feared she could still pass syphilis on to others, this woman had never again allowed herself to have a sexual relationship. She kept her highly stigmatized condition a secret. Determined that she could never marry or have children, she even distanced herself from her own family, who she believed would have rejected her if they discovered her situation.

My responsibility had only been to take her medical history and present it to the attending physician, a red-faced Friar Tuck–like figure who winked conspiratorially at me and said that I had just heard a bit of medical history about the downside of the first "magic bullet" chemotherapy.

But I still felt the humiliation and regret in that woman's tragic life story. So each week when she returned for treatments for her liver and neurological problems, she and I would talk in great detail about her past, the losses she had experienced, and her belief that the secret she had kept so devotedly had itself, more than the physical damage, ruined her life. I came to understand that our sessions meant something more to her than the various symptomatic treatments did. She told me that I was the first person to hear her full story. I learned to hear the hurt behind her words, and to recognize her heroism for what she had had to bear. I was coming to understand how the ability to enter in and work through ordinary experience itself opened a window on life and its meanings. And how the tone of a conversation, if one worked hard enough to hear it, could be part of care. When I explained to her that it was our final session, because I was rotating to another clinical specialty, she cried and whispered that our sessions had helped her to feel alive and both physically and "spiritually" better. I had discovered that meanings could heal—without being tutored or even realizing that what I was doing itself was a form of therapy. The initial patient-doctor interaction, the physical examination, the follow-up visits to deal with laboratory findings, differential diagnoses, and treatment—all can be carried out in such a way as to be therapeutic. And it is the patient as much as the doctor who makes the relationship work. That lesson has lasted and been proved true over the entire course of my career.

It was also during this period of my medical training that I began to see, through my patients, how poverty grinds down lives until they break. The fact that I was born to wealth and raised without ever concerning myself about the cost of living didn't mean that I was ignorant about poverty in the abstract. I had read enough about the Dust Bowl and heard enough about the Great Depression to know how much poverty mattered. My turn to the left in college, fueled in part by reading revolutionary socialists, gave me the theoretical understanding of, and passion for, social justice. But that understanding didn't become concrete until I witnessed the effect of poverty on my patients' lives, their social suffering. In the pediatric clinic at the Santa Clara Valley County Hospital, I met migrant Mexican American farmworker mothers and their malnourished children, and felt the outrage well up inside me. In such a rich part of such a rich country, how could there be children whose parents couldn't afford food, including some of the very foods they harvested for the tables of middle-class Americans? The pediatricians prescribed medications for the parasites and infections that resulted from the children's ravaged immune systems and their constant exposure to polluted water and high doses of pesticides. But what they needed to prescribe—and what they knew but were prohibited from doing by professional and institutional policy—was food and a less dangerous work environment.

In the emergency room, I spoke with elderly men who had been left behind by working-class families who had moved to other parts of the country in search of opportunity. These men were emaciated, often living on less than a dollar a day. They were unable to afford dental care, so their mouths were like ruins. Medicare and Medicaid were still years away at the time, so the men couldn't pay for even the most basic health care. They presented with all the classic chronic conditions of poverty: tuberculosis, infected skin wounds that had become large abscesses, and even untreated cancers, including one memorable case of a huge ulcerating tumor of the face that was no longer treatable.

As terrible as their physical conditions were, it was their shattered spirits that hit me hardest. I remember one elderly gentleman who couldn't or wouldn't look me in the eye. He mumbled that he was ashamed of his failing health, and recounted how he had poured what little money he had down his throat in the form of cheap wine. He believed that he was "not worthy"—I can still hear the words—of being treated like a decent human being. It turned out he was only in his late forties, even though he looked thirty years older.

A Spanish-speaking farmworker complained of pain in his spine, while explaining that he had to work in the fields with a hoe that was too short to allow him to stand straight as he worked and relieve the pain from bending his back all day. He came into the clinic seeking an affordable pain medication. Stupidly, I asked the interpreter to find out why the man didn't quit his job and find some other kind of work. The interpreter just looked at me without speaking, eye to eye, until the resounding silence forced me to apologize.

These experiences stayed with me. I was discovering that the social face of medicine mattered just as much as any clinical know-how I gained. The clinical years of medical school fostered in me both a rising awareness of human suffering and an appreciation of the inadequacy of medical responses to the seemingly unlimited varieties of that suffering.

The summer after my second year of medical school, a year after the powerful experiences in Alsace and Israel, I rotated through a rehabilitation medicine service at New York University's well-known Rusk Institute, where I could observe adolescents and young adults with spinal cord injuries undergoing rehabilitation. I was struck that for many of these patients, progress was in the hands of the physical therapists, more so than with the physicians, who often had little to offer in the way of medical treatment. The therapists coached patients with extremely limited movement to maximize what functions they still possessed. I learned that often, even a very small improvement in function can represent the difference between getting around and doing things independently, or giving up and retreating into complete incapacity and despair. These remarkable physical therapists plotted the parameters of success into the training programs so that even minimal change became a real achievement. They pushed, they supported, they cheered, even in the face of setbacks or failure. They entered their patients' private space and dwelled there, encouraging and remotivating those who had lost hope, moving patients out of a demoralized state of inactivity into the active, if greatly difficult, work of coping.

Years later I was assigned to lead a group therapy session for a dozen teens and young adults who had been rendered paraplegic or quadriplegic by accidents. They were all early in their experience of disability and had not had access to the kind of high-level rehabilitation services I had observed at Rusk. These patients were uniformly demoralized; still, I tried to coax them out of their negativity, naively attempting to persuade them that in time they would make peace with their disability and that neither depression nor suicide were reasonable options. Of course, they would have none of it, each one in turn declaring that indeed suicide was the only option, since they could not regain a normal body. It is with some shame that I recall their outrage, how they angrily let me know that I could never know, never understand their situation, because I did not share it. The lesson was harsh. I had foolishly tried to impose an idea of care from the outside, rather than connecting with the inner emotional lives of the recipients of care by just being there with them in their tough daily experience and struggling through the work with them.

The moral as well as the practical wisdom is that caregiving must be driven by the deepest needs of those cared for, care recipients—their pain, their anguish, their fears. The caregiver must strive to get inside the place where the care recipient exists, no matter how desolate and hopeless that place feels. Patients need to know that they will not be left alone or behind, and that you, the caregiver, are also willing to reveal your own vulnerability. It means thinking of hope as a work in progress, built and rebuilt through constant tinkering with the therapeutic regimen as the caregiver joins and also endures in the care recipient's struggle.

At the same time as I was learning the importance of making personal and emotional contact with patients, my early visits to patients' homes helped me feel my way forward among the material and personal things that make each person's experience of illness and care unique.

The first such visit was to the home of a young woman who was addicted to barbiturates. I first met her in a hospital clinic, where she was dismissed as "drug seeking" and noncompliant—a potentially difficult patient, who seemed to have little insight into her condition. My colleagues at the clinic regarded her as unreliable and uninterested in remedying her situation. The professor of preventive medicine thought I should follow up with her at home because she had such a poor record of keeping hospital appointments.

I drove to a miserable part of East Palo Alto that I hadn't even known existed, where this woman had a small apartment in a broken-down two-story building. I was surprised to see three small children living there with her. I'm not sure what I expected to find, but the apartment was clean and clearly well kept, and the children were nicely dressed and running around happily in constant play. The patient welcomed me warmly, and spoke easily and openly. Very quickly, the circumstances of her life became clear: she was a hardworking cleaner in the local middle school, and she also worked on the weekend cleaning houses on the wealthy side of town. Twice divorced, she had her small children enrolled in preschool and second grade. Virtually every waking moment of her life was devoted to work or to the apparently loving care of her children. Her barbiturate dependency resulted from problems sleeping. Rather than a difficult and demanding patient, the friendly woman I encountered in her home impressed me as a model of a self-reliant individual facing a challenging financial reality who saw the proper care of her children as her sole priority. I was shocked by the discrepancy between the way she was seen in the clinic and the way I saw her at home. Ever since, I have remained suspicious of clinical evaluations of individuals and families labeled as burdens on the health care system, unless those assessments include home visits. Too often, those descriptions represent the biases, frustrations, and blindness of clinicians to the context of their patients' human condition.

The vast majority of American medical schools today fail to provide students with adequate opportunity to observe or participate in home health care. (In the past, there were a small number, like Stanford, that did so as an elective.) Yet it is in their own homes that we see how people actually live, how they handle their illnesses or those of others, and why they might pose "problems" for health care agencies. Leiden University in the Netherlands, one of the grand old European medical schools, has had a model for teaching medical students clinical care that begins by placing beginning students in the homes of patients and families facing serious disorders. Rather than delivering traditional medical care, the students spend a week washing, cleaning, cooking, as well as performing such basic care activities as bathing, dressing, feeding, and ambulating the sick person. The goal is for the students to learn firsthand how illness is experienced and treated in the family and network, and what it feels like to join the efforts. I spoke to a number of Leiden's former students when I was invited to give a school-wide lecture there. The consensus was that this experience grounds students in family care so firmly that they are much better prepared to undertake primary care activities and much more likely to ask salient questions about family, means, caregiving, and needs. Of course, some students inevitably find the experience distasteful and discover they are not suited to this intensity of human connection and care, but better they learn that as students, with time to change direction, than as working doctors who are uncomfortable with clinical intimacy and the realities of the patient's world and needs.

Occasionally I wake up in the middle of the night with the fleeting remains of a frightening dream. The images vary, but one image in particular goes back to my days as a beginning clinical student. A small group of us were bussed to an old, crumbling state hospital, where we were led into—and then immediately fled—a crowded ward for young people with awful congenital deformities and profound cognitive impairments. I remember patients with huge hydrocephalic heads lying unresponsive in large cribs, a microcephalic man as tall as me but with a head one-third the size of mine, grinning and clapping his hands wildly, and a young man bent almost in half with a severely deformed spine,

shuffling toward me and crying out for help. Others were shouting, many
half-dressed, and the overpowering smell of urine and feces made me gag. The scene was so horrible that we medical students were moved to lodge a complaint with the state authorities about the inhuman warehousing of real people without proper care or any evidence of rehabilitation efforts, and staff acting like prison guards rather than health professionals. The complaint was never answered. Nor were we debriefed following this tormenting experience, as if our instructors had no purpose for exposing us to this clinical hell other than shocking us with the worst of care.

Inexorably, medical school changed me as it changes all aspiring physicians. I became more and more efficient at eliciting the kind of information from patients that leads to an appropriate diagnosis and useful treatment. I learned to use the tools and instruments of the profession: stethoscope, ophthalmoscope, blood pressure cuff, reflex hammer, and so on. At the same time, I honed the use of my senses as natural tools, learning to palpate, to read a pulse, to become a living gauge of pain, anxiety, depression, and so many other subjective conditions. But as my training progressed, I couldn't help feeling that I was losing touch with the sense of awe that had filled me when I held the hand of the little burn patient or spoke with the elderly woman whose life had been ruined by syphilis. I could understand that a certain professional distance was a kind of doctor's survival technique, useful for doing demanding clinical work at a high level of expertise over a long period of time. But that distancing also represented a kind of estrangement, an objectification that was neither necessary nor good. I had not gone into medicine so that I could turn away from the innermost feelings of care. My medical education had brought me to a crossroad, a crisis of value commitments.

Even as I was becoming a real doctor, a good doctor, I was developing a resistance to the destructive forces in the socialization experience the process entailed. I stopped fighting my natural instinct to reject bureaucratic indifference, professional cynicism, and self-interest. I did not want my needs as a physician in practice ever to count for more than that of my patients.

Research comparing first-year with final-year cohorts of medical students has more recently shown that my early intuition was sadly correct. Graduating students, of course, do much better than incoming students in the technical aspects of interviewing patients required for making accurate diagnoses and providing appropriate treatment. But shockingly, first-year students are better at the psychosocial, emotional, and human aspects of taking the patients' medical history. That is to say, there is something untoward, even toxic, in much of the training of doctors that undermines their social and existential skills at the same time that their technical knowledge and competencies are advancing. Half a century on, I recognize this is what I was up against and trying to resist in my medical education.

Like many medical students, I found it difficult to choose a medical specialization. At one point, I considered going into surgery. But I was most attracted to primary care internal medicine because it would make me focus on the care of patients with chronic medical conditions. That care would require getting to know patients as human beings, coming to an understanding of how their local worlds, their lives and environments, influenced the diseases and treatments, and helping them manage their conditions so that they might be able to function and feel a sense of mastery, however limited. This, I had learned, can make the critical difference in living a satisfying life. I was also interested in what at the time was called tropical medicine, and now is known as global health. Doing direct health care and prevention in poor societies appealed to my interests in diseases of poverty, in social medicine and social justice. Psychiatry also caught my interest as a way to unite my medical work with the humanities. But Stanford Medical School in the 1960s was dominated by academic researchers, basic scientists including several Nobel Prize winners, who regarded these clinical fields as lacking a clear scientific basis. We students were to be trained primarily in science, and only secondarily in the art of care.

I had begun to wonder if it was at all possible to combine the practical craft of clinical work with narratives and histories. I longed to unite the engagement with patients, their lives and communities, with my passion for ideas from what were regarded in scientific circles as the "soft" social sciences and humanities. I did find my way to a seminar in medical anthropology—the study of the social dimensions of lives, health, and illness across cultures—but it only confused and frustrated me further, failing to convincingly illuminate the work of the clinician and the public health practitioner through social theory and field research.

Hardly anyone I came across in medical school—including the professor of medical history—endorsed this interdisciplinary approach. At best, there was some halfhearted support for the most practical interventions from the social sciences that could help clinicians resolve treatment issues. But I was interested in something more: a conceptual rethinking of medicine within a larger social context. How could we better understand disease and treatments not only in individual human terms, but as problems of poverty, stigma, and culture? Only one of my teachers completely agreed and was himself a model of integrating biomedical research with social science studies. David Hamburg chaired the Department of Psychiatry, but also developed the

Program in Human Biology and collaborated on behavioral research with chimpanzees in Africa. He alone stood out as an intellectual exemplar of what I aspired to do and proof that it was realistic. David Hamburg became a lifelong mentor. He taught me that a biosocial framework was the only one that adequately addressed illness and care.

Another critical dimension to my vision was one that hardly anyone acknowledged. If care depends on the deep interaction between the caregiver and the patient, don't we need to understand the personal and social factors affecting those on either side of the relationship, so apparent to me during my medical training?

I had seen Mexican American patients, for example, who as Spanish speakers, were often poorly understood, and how neglectfully they were diagnosed and treated. Health care professionals generally appreciated the language problem but rarely took steps to correct it. More importantly, there seemed to be another part of the story that went beyond language, involving genuine differences in culture and experience. For instance, I observed several elderly Italian men who had been poisoned by wild mushrooms collected in the Santa Cruz mountains. They had mistaken a poisonous variety for one they prized. One man would go on to die of kidney failure, but two others were saved by medical interventions. One told the resident that he had every intention of going back into the woods again to search for this delicacy. The house staff expressed amazement and wrongly classified the patient as ignorant. In reality, he had made a value judgment that the staff found at best inexplicable and at worst irresponsible. He chose to risk his life in order to savor a food that in his own words was "beautiful." The doctors had no tolerance for such cultural difference in food and aesthetic preference.

An elderly Portuguese woman who was dying of end-stage

multiple sclerosis seemed unnaturally and unreasonably happy at the end of her life. For that reason, a psychiatric consult was called, on the assumption that the discrepancy between her response to death and that of the medical team, in and of itself, defined her as mentally ill. But it seemed clear enough to me that she was joyful about the prospect of meeting God very soon. And at the local Veterans Administration Hospital, I encountered two World War II veterans who had just come west for the winter and, having spent the summer and fall playing golf in New York State, were complaining because their chronic pain slowed their game. The clinic staff sniggered that they were malingerers or hypochondriacs, that their pain wasn't quite real or at least worthy of their attention. Plainly, though, these men had suffered substantial combat-related injuries and had been certified as disabled. Yet they had formed companionship and a lifestyle around their limitations, and sought relief in a medical system in order to pursue their choices. Why were we laughing at them? Why were we not treating their pain and providing rehabilitation? And if inappropriate use and misuse of health care was at issue, why weren't we dealing with it? We had no idea of their war experiences, their personal lives, or the value of golf and friendship in their lives. Was this their failure or ours? Looking back, this last instance now seems a stretch, but at the time, I was upset by the stereotyping and stigmatizing by the medical staff of men who lived with war injuries and were pursuing such exercise and pleasure as they could manage.

Even more numerous were the cases that involved ethical questions or decisions. Why had one potential recipient been chosen over another to receive a kidney? There were no rules or guidelines or computerized algorithms at the time. There was no formal process to our clinical work where a patient's treatment, or lack thereof, could be considered as an issue of health policy, ethics, or social justice. To me, the ethical issues became particularly unsettling in the cases involving medical errors that were neither admitted nor dealt with. Families that were bold enough to question the care they received usually confronted the same wall of silence. In obstetrics, a woman's stated wishes (such as Joan's) to avoid an epidural so she could feel the delivery of her child, or to be given a particular kind of anesthesia, were regularly dismissed as meddling with decisions that were not hers to make.

There was a simply huge imbalance in the doctor-patient relationship in favor of the medical professional. From the perspective of the present-day emphasis on patient education and empowerment, not to mention the ready medical advice on the Web, the accepted practices of the early 1960s seem antiquated. The world of professional dominance, or even independence, is gone forever, only to be replaced by a new set of restraints on the doctor-patient connection. But back then, I was consumed by these questions, even though I didn't know how to approach them. I was only aware of a deep and almost desperate feeling that social theory, culture, psychology, and even philosophy were somehow fundamental to the practice of medicine. I wanted to talk about how to order those factors and experiences into a systematic framework. I was asking if we could connect health care with human problems in a way that bridged the clinic with the community, the family and the society. I wanted to see field studies of doctoring that would get at the cultural worlds of practice and their impact on professionals' performance and health outcomes. It frustrated me that no one else I encountered in the clinical domain wanted to pursue these concerns. In fact, my interest was often met with cynicism, dismissed as matters beyond what anyone in clinical medicine could remedy and thus a waste of time to even consider. At the time, I could not see that this very absence would be the empty space in which I would build my career.

The sobering historical irony is that even today, when that formerly empty space has been occupied by experts in both the social sciences and medicine, and even in new fields like medical ethics and medical humanities, whose research has been presented in thousands of research articles and hundreds of books, the actual application of this sea of knowledge to clinical practice and to family care remains so limited that even my earliest thoughts, which began in medical school, are still relevant.

Three

I met my wife of nearly forty-six years just after returning from that memorable and formative summer trip to Europe, as I was transitioning away from the classroom to the clinical side of my medical education. This singular relationship—I think of it as a love story playing out over five decades—did more than anyone or anything I had encountered in my studies or in my life until then to hasten my emotional and moral awakening.

I still marvel that our relationship survived the misadventure of our first meeting. I encountered Joan completely by chance as we were both making our way to a showing of a classic French film on campus. She reminded me of one of the great stars of the day, Audrey Hepburn, in the way she looked and carried herself, and I was instantly in love. On the surface, we appeared to be opposites: me the scrappy, self-absorbed, standoffish, and intense Jewish striver from Brooklyn; Joan poised and quietly confident, affable and absorbed in others, an intoxicating mixture of natural California ease and a Continental worldliness born of her European education. I nearly blew it that very first evening, trying her patience with my insensitive and overreaching behavior— inviting her for coffee, then realizing I had an anatomy exam the next day and breaking the date, yet asking her to drive me to the anatomy building—but I soon persuaded her to give me another chance. I persevered, even against competition from far more pedigreed suitors, until Joan and I figured out that our different manners and backgrounds mattered little compared with what we shared on a deeper level—social and moral values, intellectual curiosity and commitment, and, of course, passion for each other. A year after our night at the movies, we overcame the resistance of both our families, and married.

To say that meeting Joan thoroughly reshaped my life would be a vast understatement. Our Chinese and South Asian friends have convinced me it was fated. She made my life; she made me. The twenty-four years before Joan feel like a distant era, my own prehistory. Over the nearly half century of our marriage, her face became my everyday reality. I came to internalize it to such a degree that right after Joan died, I was shocked to see my own face staring back at me from a mirror. So used to hers had I become that Joan's image had become my identity.

I remember her as a beautiful woman, refined, elegant, warm, and deeply loving. Having grown up in a white Protestant middle-class family in Palo Alto in the 1940s and '50s, and graduating from UC Berkeley and the University of Geneva in Switzerland as a scholarship student, Joan came of age just before America's women's movement took off. In an era when it was still expected that a woman's principal work would be marriage and raising children, she broke from cultural norms, as did other educated women of her generation, by living and traveling abroad. She cherished the sense of mature independence engendered in those experiences.

Joan returned from Geneva, where she had been studying for several years, to Palo Alto in 1963 for what she thought would be a transitional year, hoping to make enough money to return to

Europe for the long term. Instead, she met me. After our marriage, and as we moved between cities and countries for my training and fieldwork, she went on to study Chinese language at Yale; Chinese art history, especially painting and calligraphy, at the National Palace Museum in Taipei; to earn her MA in classical Chinese at the University of Washington in Seattle; and to become the longest-term student of the late, great sinologist Achilles Fang at Harvard. When I met Joan, she was working as a research associate of Yuan-Li Wu, a well-known economist of China at Stanford's Hoover Institute.

Joan introduced me to the Chinese aesthetic and moral traditions that she had discovered and that resonated so deeply with her. These values would become part of the foundation of our family ethos. The Chinese worldview centered on the here and now, on incorporating a moral and aesthetic responsibility into everyday life. To live a good life, you needed to cultivate the self and the relationships that made you and your world more human. For Joan, this meant creating beauty and wisdom and love in all aspects of our lives, which she accomplished through kindness, respect, reciprocity, and finding an authenticity of sharing her unique self with the world. It would take me decades to understand how important that kind of presence, alertness, and immediacy are to the practice of care.

But Joan also had an influential European side. She spoke beautiful French. It even came to inflect her English, so that many people believed her to be European. Her oldest friendships were with French families. Her culinary skills, which became impressive, were largely formed from French cookbooks and from being in the kitchen with older Frenchwomen who became surrogate mothers. It was often remarked to me, and Joan believed it herself, that her personality changed when she was speaking

French and in French surroundings. She became even more lively, imaginative, and freer with her wit and warmth. Our limited income was managed by Joan with such daily thrift that many summers we were able to visit Paris and/or the Jura mountains, where she had good friends. She rarely bought clothes, but those she did purchase came from winter or summer sales in Left Bank stores and matched the latest fashion. When not reading Chinese texts, she read classic French literature, especially the great essayists like Chateaubriand and Montaigne, as well as the novels of Balzac, Zola, and Proust. *Poulet à l'estragon* was her go-to dish for dinners at our home, as was her Franco-American upside-down apple-crisp version of *tarte Tatin*. When we were in Paris we would walk for up to an hour before she found a restaurant suitably interesting yet inexpensive.

In raising our children, she emphasized their learning of both Chinese and French language and culture. From the French tradition, she took a deep appreciation of style, quality, and seriousness about crafting elegance in living. I also attributed her precise diction and precision in most things to her French experience. But she wore these values so lightly they never seemed forced or affected. "Natural" is the best word for the way these various elements were embodied in her.

Joan took care of the aesthetic, religious, and moral sides of our marriage and family. Her kindness, decency, and ready smile were genuine and understated, and served as a model of authenticity and goodness for our children and for me. As much as moral values mattered to her, she was not a moralizer, and she was downright suspicious of those who were. She believed in God as a force in the world, but not in institutionalized religion or theology. She read the Bible regularly, but she prayed to the God of a plural, diverse universe and enjoyed religious stories of all kinds.

At the core of her way of being, though, were the good words and good acts that mattered to people in the practical world she inhabited. They sanctified the world.

She gave a very great deal of thought and attention to the details of the everyday activities of our lives from an ordinary weeknight dinner to family holidays and parties for friends. She knew that the simple addition of candles could transform an everyday meal into an event and a celebration. She encouraged liveliness and depth in our conversations, and organized family readings of classics, insisting that each of us read our portion with gusto and expression. Joan made the most delicious and elegant picnics—roast chicken or rice salad, barbecued ribs, her tarte Tatin, an interesting cheese, a good wine, with lemonade or sparkling water for the kids. These meals would be set out on a Provençal tablecloth placed over a Chinese bamboo mat with cloth napkins, our best cutlery, and real plates, no matter if we were at the Tanglewood Music Festival or a state park. Joan had not come from money, and in the early years of our marriage, our finances were stretched thin, so these rituals were the product of careful intention and self-discipline. The message was as important as the meal: there is a way to do things that elevate life to be more cultivated and meaningful. Joan was a master artisan; life was her medium.

Joan expressed harmony and balance in her way of living. She moved seamlessly between her Chinese calligraphy and painting, her masterly gardening, her French and Chinese cooking, and her dedicated, immersive child-rearing, while always finding time to celebrate and nurture our most intimate relationship as a couple. She led us on family walks in the countryside, taught us to identify trees and feel their spirited presence, and made sure we played sports together. Everything Joan did for us knit us closer together as a family. Even Salty, our large, unruly dog, mellowed in her presence.

I remember one episode that defined not only her compassion and courage but also her steely determination. When I was in the midst of my internal medicine internship at the Yale New Haven Hospital—a full year (June 1967–June 1968) in which I was in the hospital twenty-four hours followed by a twelve-hour day and every other weekend—my fellow intern took ill, forcing me to work in the hospital for five nights in a row. Midway through that impossible time, Joan called me in the night to tell me that our son, Peter, who was then seven months old, had a fever of 107 degrees. She had called the pediatrician, who told her it was probably rubella and that anyway he was too busy to make a home visit. I was tremendously angry at the hospital and the pediatrician, but I couldn't leave the hospital. I was responsible for patients all around me with life-threatening illnesses. Joan gave Peter ice baths and eventually brought down his fever. Through it all, she was calm but alert and fiercely effective, whereas I was beside myself with fear, anguish, and guilt.

That same trying year, I underwent my own quiet personal crisis. I had started to feel that my mind was drying up. On the alternating nights when I was at home, Joan would cook a meticulously prepared and delicious dinner, but I would often ignore or even reject her meal in order to sit alone and read something outside of medicine to keep my mind alive. Recognizing how desperate I was to devote time to my intellectual passion, she would go along with my selfish desire and support my needs. And over the years to come I learned to reciprocate. But while I supported her passion for studies in language and art history, I could not match what she did for me, leaving her disappointed and me guilty.

In 1976 we relocated to Seattle, where I took a tenured post at the University of Washington. My stepfather died that year, and my mother seemed to become unmoored. Joan suggested we invite her to leave New York and come live with us, believing the kids needed to have a grandparent nearby. I was hesitant; my relationship with my mother had become distant. I feared she would be a burden, maybe even a divisive force in the family. Joan insisted, though, and so I extended the invitation. Responding to Joan's and the kids' encouragement, my mother bravely moved out to Seattle, a city she had never even visited. Joan found her a perfect place to live and diligently engineered opportunities for her to develop a very close relationship with our children, where previously there had been only distance. She and Joan became great friends, and I developed a less complicated, freer relationship with my mother than I had ever had. For her part, my mother had the chance to reinvent herself as a grandmother, drawing on her inner strength and resourcefulness. This renewed relationship changed her life and it contributed centrally to ours. It could not have happened without Joan.

During those six years in Seattle and continuing after we returned to Cambridge, my health deteriorated. I developed sinusitis, asthma, hypertension, and gout. No doubt these problems were largely of my own making. I swung between near-manic periods of hyperproductive work during which I slept little, and crashing hard, having to take to bed, symptomatic and exhausted. Joan, who was, amazingly, always in superb health, would tend to me as if she had another child in her care.

Things reached a breaking point in 1980, while our family was spending five months in Changsha, the capital of Hunan Province in China—the first Americans to live there since 1949. It was a blistering summer, with stifling humidity and daytime temperatures reaching 110 degrees. In the Chinese faculty housing where we lived, for the first month we only had two small electric fans. The water pressure was so low that we couldn't shower but only bathe in a few inches of tepid water. We all developed heat rashes, like our Chinese colleagues, who occasionally slept outside, hoping to feel the little breeze coming off the river. Despite the difficult living conditions, I was determined to finish research on a hundred patients, all victims of the Cultural Revolution, who suffered from the symptoms of "neurasthenia"—fatigue, pain, dizziness, anxiety, and demoralization. This research was extraordinarily demanding, but it would make my name in Chinese psychiatry for introducing the modern idea of depression and its treatment there (and in the United States, too, for my work on the relationship of political trauma and culture to psychiatry). As summer ended, Joan and the children returned to the United States for the school year, but I had a month more to go with fifteen cases left to finish.

Left on my own, I developed dysentery and some gruesome complications, along with a crisis of my asthma and overall poor condition. I lost 20 percent of my body weight in those weeks, and all confidence in my health. And still I persisted in completing the research. My Chinese friends worried that I might not survive. When I returned to Seattle, Joan and the children could scarcely recognize me. It took months to recover, but Joan was fierce in her efforts to care for this broken man. She pulled me through.

She was there for me again a year later when I awoke from a nightmare in absolute panic. Sweat poured down my face, my heart raced, and I could barely catch my breath. Joan calmed me, and listened as I recounted my terrible dream. I was in harness pulling a heavy chariot through the sky. The charioteer whipped me to go faster and faster, until finally, I stopped and yelled that I could not go faster. Out of breath and angry, I turned around to confront the merciless charioteer, but I was shocked to see that the man holding the reins and the whip was me. My asthma took hold of me and I was helplessly gulping for air as Joan and I tried to make sense of the nightmare. I remember breaking down and weeping. "I need you, I need you, I need you now," I gasped. Joan turned herself over to caring for me, slowly, imperceptibly, re-building my confidence over the months that passed. We were together, bonded, pulling in the same direction, loving, as I began the long, slow process of remaking myself. I was attempting to care for my own body and soul, maybe for the first time. I was damaged, and could not have come through it alone. It was be-cause I trusted Joan so completely that I could finally allow myself to be fully vulnerable. She saved me. It was as simple as that.

On a few rare occasions during those early years of our mar-riage, I found Joan crying quietly. She told me that she felt a deep sadness at times, which she related to never having bonded closely with her own mother. That raw spot in her own experience spurred her to create the strongest ties with her children and with me and also with her mother-in-law, whom she always called "Mother." My mother responded in kind, telling me and others that Joan was the daughter she had never had but always yearned for.

We had our bad moments, as couples do, for in many ways we were yin and yang, complementary opposites. These rough patches were usually on me: my failures by being absent when the children were young; my insufficient support for Joan when she was balancing graduate school and family life; the total absorp-tion in my work that made me "a drudge," "inattentive," and "un-inspiring," as she would put it. I knew when she was annoyed with me, because on those occasions she would call me with emphasis

"Arthur Michael" in place of "Arthur." When she was genuinely angry she could be fierce, but in a silent mode. She looked hard in my eyes—no smile, no softness, no words. Twice, she reached across for my eyeglasses, and without saying anything, slowly crushed them in her hand. These failures we each remembered. But these were, with several exceptions, fleeting and part of the flow of our lives.

Joan created a special world for me and our children, Peter and Anne. We were enveloped by an atmosphere of golden warmth and cultivation that we came to take for granted, as did our wider family, friends, colleagues, and students. We eventually understood that Joan had built a solid foundation that would support our long-term future after its creator had passed on. Her unspoken lesson was that this special world could not be simply assumed, but had to be crafted each day.

Early in our career as collaborators in China research, Joan set a pattern with students and colleagues: I would oversee the academics, while she looked after our scholarly ties and relationships, a function she took to be as critical as the academic work itself. Blunt and often undiplomatic in scholarly affairs, I was not easy, in my thirties and forties, for students to approach directly. Many hesitated; some actually cowered, genuinely frightened of me. They preferred to communicate with me through Joan, who could advocate for them. Even colleagues, especially Chinese and European colleagues, felt more comfortable in those early years speaking with Joan, particularly about some of the more contentious issues that our research generated. As if her comparative warmth and emotional openness weren't enough, her Chinese, like her French, was much better than mine, making them feel that they were better understood by her.

Joan prioritized the care of relationships and embracing their emotional and moral consequences. Our colleagues and students recognized this, and reserved their warmest feelings for her. They may have valued me as a mentor and an intellectual interlocutor, but in Joan they valued humanity. The Chinese call this quality *ren*, and Chinese friends often talked about Joan as someone who knew how to create and sustain *renqinq guanxi*—cultivated moral relationships. I fully understood why they saw this in Joan, because I did, too, even as I had to acknowledge that they didn't feel the same way about me. I knew that the real achievement belonged to her, because her positive effect on people went beyond the scholarly world. I paraded my knowledge in journals and from lecterns, but Joan's wisdom pervaded life itself.

Her friendships were global. Swedish, French, Swiss, and Chinese women, whom she had met at Berkeley, Geneva, later Stanford, and the University of Washington, brought her into their families, and those friendships with time came to include me and, in two special cases, our children and grandchildren. Several of these close friends would be present at Joan's bedside in her final days.

Through long and intimate letters and telephone calls she responded to important events in these families—weddings, births, new jobs, but also crises and deaths. So that decades before Face-Time, social media, and Skype, we were connected in a vital network of mutually supportive relationships. Joan worked at sustaining and deepening these ties through gift exchanges, extended visits, and always managing to be present when friends truly needed her.

But even in everyday relations with co-workers, neighbors, and the staff of nearby shops, as well as with the electricians, plumbers, and handymen whom she hired to fix household problems, Joan had an effect on people that built trust and meaning.

From a crusty old housepainter to the bashful Brazilian immigrants (probably some undocumented) who cleaned our house, to a worn older woman at the supermarket checkout counter, I heard the respect they had for her, and for the attention she paid to their personal situations. She did more than smile and remember their names; she made it her business to know who they were and what they were facing. Not infrequently, she was there to help by listening, translating official documents, making calls on their behalf to their banks, insurance companies or government offices, and calming their anguish. More than a few of these workers, whom I hardly knew, would attend her memorial service.

Over the years, I learned from Joan to refashion my academic relationships and my way of being with others. I came to see that a warm smile, a responsive greeting, and a genuine thank-you acknowledges the other person, affirming who they are and who I am. I allowed myself to reveal my own vulnerabilities, and to be open with details of my life even when they didn't put me in a good light. I learned about life something I had earlier learned about the practice of medicine: to listen; I learned to respond to what mattered to others. I believe simple changes to my behavior made me more human, more sympathetic and approachable. Although learned, as these became habits they made me a different person. I could feel myself shedding my defensive armor and the overweening aspiration that had weighed me down. I could feel a lightening of the spirit within that increased my happiness and eased the tension in my more fraught relationships. Surely my clinical work, the natural maturation that comes with age, and the experiences of parenting and mentoring were factors in my evolution, but I know now that by learning how to tend to these relationships in ways both big and small, I was really learning to tend to myself. As after my earlier physical collapse, Joan was the effective agent of change; her presence softened me and, at the same time, opened up new ways for me to be me. She became my innermost model of how to live life.

Joan Kleinman healed me—slowly, but progressively, over decades. She trained me to take care, be careful, and give care. The consequence of the transformation in me was an expansive and inclusive happiness. I came to regard my family life as golden. The times were joyful and we looked ahead with great expectations.

The new kind of engagement also infused my academic and professional work. My research emphasis turned from cognitive aspects of disease pathology and treatment to the emotional and moral sides of the lived experience of pain and disablement. Personal histories with fuller engagement of subjectivity and context now took precedence for me over quantitative assessments of distress and disease. The new definitions and models of cultural systems of health care that had characterized my early publications now gave way to stories: illness narratives by patients and healers. My writing style followed the change in methods. The labored and pressurized scientific language surrendered to freer and more emotionally evocative descriptions of real lives. One perceptive foreign critic praised it as an example of the feminization of my writing. Over time, my teaching also became less technical and more existential. I developed new courses, and purposely gave them long and evocative names such as Biography, Ethnography, the Novel, Film and Psychotherapy: Deep Ways of Knowing the Person in the Social Context; Deep China: The Emotional and Moral Person. Later still I taught Quests for Wisdom: Religious, Moral and Aesthetic Experiences in the Art of Living with co-instructors Davíd Carrasco, Michael Puett, and Stephanie Paulsell. These replaced courses with dry, technical names for specific topics in medical anthropology, cultural psychiatry, global mental health, and social medicine. The direction was clear: from specialized technical knowledge to more generalized human knowledge, from abstract ideas to moral experiences of real people and what mattered most to them.

Joan took a formal role in the research projects, partly so that we could spend more time together, but her very presence transformed studies of the diagnosis and treatment of depression and specific medical disorders into studies of the experiences of pain, fatigue, and demoralization in the broad context of families, communities, and society as a whole. She insisted on moral interpretations of research findings that illuminated their existential significance.

Even my clinical teaching took this turn. Clinical rounds that had been called psychiatric consultation rounds or clinical medical anthropology rounds became moral, cultural, and psychosocial rounds or simply Kleinman rounds. The latter incorporated all of my efforts to humanize medical practice. I co-taught courses on religion and medicine with Sarah Coakley and later still on the medical humanities with David Jones and Karen Thornber.

My clinical practice in the late 1970s and '80s became less centered on medications and more on psychotherapy, working out my own unique approach, which I thought of as ethnographic psychotherapy. From more formal concerns with the interpretation of early-life conflicts and their influence on patients' current symptoms, my orientation loosened up and refocused on a shared understanding for what was most at stake in the ordinary moments of patients' lives. I no longer saw the diagnosis and treatment of depression as the end point of my practice, but as a necessary first step in understanding and repairing a deeper life process. And this happened as the profession of psychiatry took the opposite turn toward neuroscience, making me stand out as either an anachronistic throwback to the days of healers or a portent of a new era where psychiatry meant high-quality care.

I could join my patients in exploring the meanings of care in their experiences and look for sources of wisdom that were useful in their lives and in my own. My relationships with my patients became more reciprocal and egalitarian. We were all in this together, sharing the risk, the appreciation of incompleteness, the fragments of memory, and the brokenness of life that are the prerequisite to healing. This last resoundingly fell into place later, when I myself became a family caregiver.

At about the time this transformation was occurring, I had a patient who was a writer for a small newspaper in a coastal fishing port. He had a drinking problem, coupled with chronic depression. His marriage was in trouble, but what made him most desperate was the confidence-undermining feeling that he would remain trapped, writing forever for this little-read paper. He believed he had astonishing stories to tell, stories that he felt could make his name and career. All he needed was to somehow muster the energy and discipline to get them out of his fragile psyche and published in large-circulation journals and newspapers where they could attract the big readership he believed they deserved. A tall, bearded, handsome man, who was about my own age, this patient fluctuated between bouts of high confidence, usually when he was drinking, and hopelessness when he was sober. I was able to reverse his depressed symptoms and, for a while at least, help him control his drinking behavior. In the past, this would have been enough because it satisfied my understanding of what I needed to do as his psychiatrist. But I permitted myself to address the camaraderie I felt with him. As a writer myself I had the same hope and aspiration. Indeed I experienced the same pang of regret for not yet writing the kind of work that would bring me wider recognition. And so together we explored this shared dilemma. My family's cross-country move cut short the treatment, and I never learned whether our mutual exploration of this problem led to an improved outcome. But as a caregiver, I felt more comfortable and optimistic having shared our mutual tribulation and having tried to make useful sense out of what we both could imagine was a much larger existential theme. I know I benefited from recognizing myself as a wounded healer, long after the sharp outline of this case blurred in my memory.

Slowly but increasingly, I learned to be more open and responsive to my students as well. Early in my career, graduate students and medical students had commanded most of my attention, but now I turned more and more to undergraduates as the primary object of my teaching. I sensed that with these younger students, I could more readily explore the broadest range of issues that mattered to me most—and, I hoped, to them. In fact, it was only through teaching—having to organize and communicate the ideas that now consumed my thinking—that I clearly identified these themes. I discovered that they paralleled so much of what I had already written about: the slow transformation in my soul. It was *experiences* that I wished to explore and shape—experiences of pain, injury, and suffering and their makeover in therapy and care—and how to approach these as a healer and a writer. In my vision, experience combined social and personal states. Hence suffering was social as well as psychological and the most effective interventions were also both. At the same time, I sought to explore the experiences of the healer from the inside. What did healers need, in order to be more effective and to persevere while protecting themselves from burnout? Yet once again, how did the intertwined collective and individual sides of those experiences make them more powerful?

So much of this awakening was born in my experiences in China and elsewhere in the world. The cultural comparisons that emerged from our lived experience and from our research and reading altered my perspective in so many ways. I know in my heart, though, that I was able to recognize and absorb those lessons only because of Joan. She liberated me, making me ready for and attentive to new experience, not through lectures or instruction, but simply by letting her grounded, compassionate persona stand as a living example. Her relationships with others convinced me of their power in caring and mentoring. And through the quality of the relationship with me she continued to revise and reaffirm the person I was becoming.

Like the rest of us, Joan was complex. For example, she had a sharp and dry wit, to which those who sat next to her at academic seminars can testify. She openly acknowledged and affirmed everyone she spoke with, and yet in her own mind she held critical views about ideas and people. She might or might not express these, but they were there. Pretension and hypocrisy bothered her greatly, still she held her own counsel so that you might not hear her critical views unless you were personally close to her and someone she believed she could confide in. When we were out eating a fine meal or at home doing the same, she would share her portion freely with the children and me. The one exception was chocolate. A chocolate dessert was something she guarded fiercely.

After her death, several of her women friends wrote to me explaining how important Joan had been in their lives. She was a trusted confidante to many younger women, and she held their secrets so closely that I had no idea what they concerned, even when those women were colleagues, students, or my own assistants. She knew that women in her time had often been poorly and shamefully treated in academia by male supervisors and colleagues. Her own academic ambitions had been deferred in support of my career. She advocated for young women with conviction in academia. There was something in her persona so balanced and agreeable that colleagues often told me that her mere presence could lighten their mood. Her smile was infectious; no matter how down you felt, you smiled back and shared her warmth. "Warmed by the sun," one friend called it. One of the workmen she hired told me, "Your wife is so positive, you want to do anything you can for her."

When colleagues or students were sick or injured, Joan stepped right in and helped them in direct and practical ways. She mediated tense relationships between students and their families. Friends in our network sought her out for practical advice concerning troubled marriages, difficulties in parenting, and personal problems. I was the psychiatrist, but she was the network caregiver. At times I felt jealous, even as I recognized how petty that was. I realized I wanted her all to myself, but everybody appreciated Joan for who she was and what she did for others. Upon her death, it was not just me who cried, but almost everyone around me. Virtually everyone we knew believed themselves to be one of Joan's close friends.

Four

My first visit to Taiwan, in 1969, filled me with shock and wonderment. Nothing could have prepared me for the onslaught of unfamiliar sensations. The sights and sounds and smells, and the chaotic hurly-burly of the street life, were easy to get used to, however, compared with the social and cultural orientation and practices that would, over time, fundamentally alter my perspective on human interaction. After fifty years of studying Chinese society, including seven and a half years of living in Taiwan and China, I can say that I'm still learning how to parse the surface differences and similarities to get at the deeper meanings.

So many of us associate China with literal and figurative walls. I recall one day, on the drive back from a visit to a leprosarium, I asked the taxi driver why the government had built this facility on the other side of a mountain behind a high wall so far outside Taipei.

"You know Chinese views, don't you? This illness can harm people. It is caused by evil spirits. Something must block them. Distance, walls, and mountains can do that."

The notion that the unseen world is teeming with negative forces and energies, hungry ghosts, belligerent gods, and unappeased ancestors, all of which could derail your life and alter your fate, was very much alive in Taiwan in 1969. People commonly put up high walls outside and painted screens inside the house to deflect and deter these unseen forces. (They topped those walls with broken glass or barbed wire to keep out a more practical threat, burglars.) Many turned to geomancy (a process of divination based on patterns in the landscape), hoping to tap into vital power running through the ground, which could enhance one's inner life force (*qi*) and bring good fortune to the family. Others offered up prayers and rituals to placate ancestors, who might undermine the living just as readily as they would assist them. Some sought out local shamans to perform exorcisms. These rituals and practices were believed to be palpable, practical means of defining, confronting, and somehow mastering the tangible risks and dangers of the world.

Even the language I use to describe these powerful forces and the human responses to them has a kind of normalizing effect, masking how alien it all seemed to me, how much it contradicted everything I thought I knew. Add our politically correct fear of "othering" people whose culture differs from ours and you find yourself latching on to superficial similarities that hide more than they reveal.

In the 1960s American men were subject to the military draft. I had originally come to Taiwan to fulfill my Selective Service commitment, dispatched by the National Institutes of Health to serve as a US Public Health Service clinical fellow working with US Naval Medical Research Unit No. 2. The unit had a strong research tradition in infectious diseases, but was also, at the height of the Vietnam War, the backup laboratory for the US Marines hospital in Da Nang, in Vietnam. I spent most of my time there carrying out field research in both rural and urban settings, with patients suffering highly stigmatized conditions, like leprosy and tuberculosis.

Shortly after arriving in Taiwan, I traveled high into the central mountains to Wushe with a pathologist from the same unit. An Episcopal missionary had set up a church there to attempt to serve the impoverished local aboriginal community. (The aboriginal Australo-Malay population—the original inhabitants of Taiwan—had been driven into the highlands by the Chinese immigrants who occupied the fertile farming areas in the lowlands.) My colleague and I set up a medical clinic there, and for two days tended to people who had never had biomedical care. Hundreds lined up to be examined, but we were woefully ill equipped to attend to their needs.

We even got out to do some home visits, and in one small village we came to a wooden farmhouse, behind which we found a middle-aged woman living in filth with inadequate clothing, confined in a cage. The family had locked her up in this way for two reasons: her history of chronic mental illness, and a tumor in her mouth that impaired her speech and was so large we could see it when she smiled. Shocked and appalled, we tried desperately to explain that she clearly had cancer, and what she needed was treatment, not isolation. But her family shot back that they lived in fear of her madness and her tumor, which they believed were caused by sorcery that might also affect them if they allowed her to get too close.

I felt the deepest sadness for all of them, and on a more intellectual level felt outrage at the cruel injustice. I promised myself to work toward ending such abusive practices. The missionary priest took me aside and recounted how he had pleaded with the family for months to release the woman, but to no effect. It was my most direct confrontation to date with the idea that the caregiving response itself could dehumanize a person in the throes of serious suffering.

In the clinic, in a triage-like setting, we saw patients with conditions that might have been treatable at an earlier time, but who had gone for so long without professional health care that there was no longer much that could be done to help them. Given the overwhelming number of patients, the priest barely had time to translate their complaints, let alone elicit any kind of meaningful illness narrative. Barring the few obvious and acute problems I could help with, I was totally unable to deal with chronic disease in the absence of adequate medical histories, records, lab tests, and treatment options. With only a few minutes to see each patient, and access to so few treatments, I began to doubt if the clinic had any value. And yet, even here, in what physician-anthropologist Paul Farmer would later call a "clinical desert," the care had meaning. Villager after villager thanked us, profusely and sincerely, for looking at their problems, and at least trying to help. What specific meaning they drew out of the experience baffled me, but it suggested that the symbolic power physicians radiated can be more important than practical results, and that these terribly poor people were just grateful for any semblance of treatment.

In 1970, my work took me away from Taiwan briefly, to Manila, in the Philippines, where I would have another formative experience. An epidemic of cholera had broken out there, and I was ordered to a hospital in a poor section of the city to help with a treatment study. I worked twenty-four hours on, followed by twenty-four hours off, for a solid month, treating cholera patients, first with intravenous fluids, then oral fluids, to rehydrate them. Treating cholera with adequate IVs, nurses, and antibiotics was unlike anything I experienced in a clinical setting before or since. Patients of all ages arrived near death—prostrate, semiconscious, and often with a barely palpable pulse. Because of the rapid onset of explosive diarrhea, they had lost much of their body fluid, reducing their blood volume so greatly that they would soon die without intravenous fluids. Amazingly to me, once an IV had been started, the replacement fluids helped them fairly quickly to sit up, even walk, and drink on their own. With oral rehydration solutions and antibiotics, they could usually leave the hospital within a day or two. Health professionals liken the treatment of cholera to the experience of Lazarus in the Bible, coming back from the dead. Without proper medical support, though, cholera has a death rate of between 30 and 40 percent.

One case from our time in Manila still haunts me. A woman came running into the clinic, carrying an apparently lifeless six-year-old boy in her arms. I couldn't find a pulse, but I could hear the faintest of heartbeats through the stethoscope. I knew we had to act immediately before this child succumbed. We had to rehydrate him, but I couldn't find a vein on his frail limbs for an IV. Now in my hyperfocused "intern in the ER" mode, I realized the only hope was to insert a thin tube into the boy's abdomen and infuse him directly with fluids, a procedure I had never before performed.

When the boy's mother saw what I intended to do, she started yelling at me while she reached out to protect her son. The seasoned Filipino nurse explained that the mother's faith forbade injections, but at the same time, implored me to do something to save the boy's life if I could. Training and instinct took over. I grabbed the child and had the nurse take the mother away to the other side of the curtain that separated the boy's cot from the rest of the ward. I desperately pushed the tube into his abdomen and started the flow of saline solutions. Less than ten minutes later, his inert body started moving; in another fifteen minutes, he was sitting up and I was able to get an IV into his arm. Truly a Lazarus effect.

When the nurse brought the mother back in, she took the boy in her arms, thanked the nurse profusely, but only glared at me. I believe that she understood that my actions had saved her son's life, but she could not forgive my egregious violation of her belief system. Time has given me perspective on this episode. I had saved a life, but in doing so, had negated virtually everything I believe today about professional caregiving. I had acted without parental consent, while explaining almost nothing to the parent. I had shown disrespect for the family's religious principles. At the time, my only thought was to save the boy's life, and I might very well do the same thing today in such extreme circumstances. It would take me some time to process this experience as my understanding of the practice of care evolved, but I know now that by prioritizing objective clinical medicine while ignoring other concerns that mattered to a patient's family, I had acted with exactly the same kind of detached professional arrogance that would often upset and frustrate Joan and me. It is one thing to do this with acute life-threatening disease, but another thing altogether with chronic illness.

As far out of my experience as these situations were, they were not what ultimately upended my worldview. My assumptions about how the world worked were challenged more by less exotic yet more fundamental distinctions. First, I had to absorb the Chinese cultural view that we are not born fully human, that our humanity exists on a kind of spectrum or continuum. Thus, a baby is not a complete human being, and women occupy their own unique but inferior position on that spectrum. The positive manifestation is the idea that human beings need to cultivate their humanity over the course of a lifetime, an idea that fosters self-education and good habits. On the more troubling side, it justifies infanticide and potentially damaging corporal punishment of young children, as well as treatment of women as somehow lesser humans.

Second, and with greater impact on me, I learned that one's personhood is largely defined by relationships within one's family and social networks. The individual is expected not to be so singular, nor independent, but more collective. Indeed, these relationships are paramount. Almost all your hours are to be spent with others. Your needs and desires are less important than those of the group. You must learn to express yourself through family and friendship ties. Not every group matters, nor is the larger group the most important. Rather, your values are family- and network-specific. So, if a small child is wandering around lost on a busy road, the family, not strangers, are responsible. Hence you don't intervene for people unconnected to you. (From then until now, this overly narrow ethical framing is one I can't accept.)

And third, I learned that local meanings, and not universal truths, govern how we feel and interpret taste, beauty, and even goodness. What was at stake for people locally in Taiwan—their networks of relationships, their moral and religious orientations—was different from what was most at stake for me. Because of this, I could participate in, but never fully belong to, their local worlds, nor they to mine.

These unfolding revelations dovetailed with the research that had brought me to Taiwan, through which I sought to compare the treatments given to patients by biomedical physicians (the science-based practice associated with Western medicine) with those given by practitioners of traditional Chinese medicine and religious healers, such as fortune-tellers and shamans. I found that all these healers combined accounted for less than a quarter of the care provided to people experiencing illness. Families provided most of the care, in conjunction with the people who were ill themselves. This paralleled research results from the United States and elsewhere, which showed that in cultures across the world, families overwhelmingly shoulder the burden of caregiving.

As I dug deeper into how the illness experience differed depending on the healing practice, I found that the biomedical physicians generally spent less time with patients and tended to engage only on the most superficial and mechanical level with those patients. They provided minimal explanations of diagnoses and treatments and didn't want to answer a lot of questions. And they also showed little respect for patient preferences and the troubles experienced by family carers. In contrast, the relationships that patients and families had with traditional Chinese medicine practitioners were longer and warmer, and imbued with a spirit of mutual respect. These practitioners shared popular ideas about foods as medicine, traditional exercises, and therapeutic herbs and teas with their patients and their families, and related them to *qi*, *yin/yang*, and other orienting cultural principles. The family context of care, not surprisingly, was the most intimate of all, and alive with presence and shared values.

In my research with an epidemiologist, it became evident that not just in cases of chronic illness but also in situations where the symptoms defied medical explanation (suggesting they were caused by psychological or social stressors), the quality of care was highest among family, traditional practitioners, and religious healers. Biomedical practitioners, even senior ones, provided the lowest-quality care. Most importantly, the outcomes of the former were better than those of the latter too. I became deeply interested in this process of somatization, or embodiment, in which bodily symptoms without any clear-cut biological pathology can impede normal life for patients, and can result from depression, anxiety, and problems in the workplace or home. It is a subject I have worked on for five decades.

Joan and I found ourselves coming to terms with these unfamiliar perspectives in all kinds of unexpected ways. I had a friend who was a leading Taiwanese public health expert who had trained in the United States and had worked all over the world in what we would now call global public health. I went to visit him after he developed a rapidly growing cancer, but his family cautioned me not to mention the word cancer nor to speak to him about his treatment. All the clinically relevant decisions fell to the family, rather than to my friend, even though he himself was an accomplished physician. He acted as if he knew nothing about his treatment. He told me it was best not to talk about these things, because his family members had taken over complete responsibility for his care. Even at that time, this was an extreme example of the dominance of relationships over the individual person in Chinese society. Today the individual has a much larger voice, although relationships with family and friends still orient a person's life.

Other unfamiliar practices also arose out of the primacy of relationships and interactions: The bargaining that was expected over even minor items in markets and stores; the second families and minor wives who were the vestiges of a bygone polygynous society; the extreme devotion to educational achievement as the major vehicle for social upward mobility and wealth (even when viewed from an American Jewish perspective) and the high status it could confer on one's family. These practices were not the same for the poor as they were for the elite. Social class was like caste—an almost biological marker carried with you across the generations. A person you met would announce himself as the sixth generation of scholars, or the fifth generation of doctors. People accepted their status, and nobody made any pretense of caring about social inequality. The poor were disregarded or badly treated and expected nothing, more or less. Philanthropy was uncommon, as people would only give help to family and friends. Strangers were out of luck. Life among elite mainlanders in Taiwan in 1969 opened our eyes to why China had been such fertile ground for a Communist revolution.

Politics, national and cultural identity, and the indelible memories of a complex and violent history pervaded the collective consciousness of Taiwan. The island had been settled by Chinese hundreds of years earlier but had become part of the Japanese empire for the first half of the twentieth century. Japanese language and culture dominated until the end of World War II, during which the Taiwanese fought as part of Japan. With Japan's defeat, Taiwan came under the control of the Republic of China, which forcibly, brutally, put down a rebellion on the island in 1947. When Mao and the Communist Revolution overtook China two years later, Chiang Kai-shek and his Nationalists fled to Taiwan, which they ruled with an iron hand. These "mainlanders" became the ruling elite, lording their power and privilege over the 90 percent of the population who considered themselves native Taiwanese.

Political tensions and historical resentments continued to animate everyday interactions when Joan and I arrived in Taiwan, twenty years after the revolution and civil war. The authoritarian mainlander governing elite still dominated, and it was dangerous to speak out publicly about any serious matter. Many of our older acquaintances, who had retreated with the Nationalist government and army from the mainland, clung to a fierce hatred of the Japanese for what they had done to China. These mainlanders were connoisseurs whom Joan had befriended at the Palace Museum, where she studied, or they belonged to other elite circles into which she had been introduced. My friends, in contrast, were the young physicians and nurses at National Taiwan University Hospital, almost all of whom were native Taiwanese. The ones who came from educated backgrounds spoke Japanese with their parents, who had been raised to speak Japanese and to feel as if they themselves were Japanese.

This division in our friendship networks sensitized Joan and me to the central fault line cracking Taiwan in the 1960s and '70s. Neither Joan nor I had been politically active in our own country. In Taiwan, we felt the full force of history creating political oppression that we could not simply witness without acting. I was deeply impressed by my Taiwanese co-workers, who desperately wanted independence, yet felt the political tension between educated Taiwanese families who still valued the influence of Japanese culture, and the elite mainlanders who still hated the Japanese for invading China and killing more than twenty million Chinese. We sided with the Taiwanese underdogs, and lent assistance where we could. We felt like spies among the mainlander elite. We knew, too, that people were almost certainly keeping their eyes on us.

The many long years of imperial Chinese, Japanese colonial, and mainlander domination had left a mark on the psyche and behavior of the Taiwanese people. For example, the ability to endure danger and hardship—political, economic, medical—had become a cornerstone cultural trait that drove many personal interactions. I witnessed countless examples of elders who put the family first before their own health and welfare; wives who put up with vexing in-laws, co-wives, and mistresses so that their children would have a better future; and individuals who postponed their own personal aspirations in order to maintain harmony. People cultivated the family and social networks, and expressed love and care indirectly through actions, not words. You did not say "I love you." Rather, you showed love in the meals you prepared, the careers you enabled, the travel you arranged, or the tutorials you financed. The idea of love itself was not about a spontaneous feeling, the fleeting, ephemeral nature of which could not be trusted. Love and care consisted instead of a long-term commitment to strengthening ties, worrying about the family's future, and tending to its members as assiduously as you would prune bonsai trees or feed the koi in the house's small pond. Indeed, love was virtually synonymous with care, and such care made you and the family more human. In a closely connected social circle, that meant being worthy of care oneself, and at the same time responsible for caring for the others around you. One did not speak of care, just as one did not speak of love, but practiced it as an everyday ideal worth pain and effort, loyalty and courage. In fact, there is not one but many words (and word combinations) in the Chinese language for care, often connoting different ways of enacting care. Care could mean control, stewardship, caretaking, protection, caregiving, serious attention to detail, dealing with something, worry and anxiety, among other shades of meaning that are as various as in English.

Over the coming years, our family would develop bonds to mainland China, as strong as those to Taiwan. In 1980, as I described in chapter 3, Joan and I, with Peter and Anne, now thirteen and nine, respectively, spent five months at the Hunan

Medical College over an exceptionally hot summer. After Joan and the children returned to the United States, I developed dysentery, which cascaded into a traumatic, life-threatening health crisis.

I had lost so much weight I could barely keep my pants from falling down as I said goodbye to colleagues and friends. One of the Chinese academic physicians I had come to know well, a senior professor of psychiatry, said to me, "Your health is bankrupt! You know how to give care professionally, but you don't know how to care for yourself!" He was right. From that time onward—from age thirty-nine until now—I have worked harder at self-care.

Joan's committed caregiving made my ultimate recovery possible, but that couldn't have happened without my devoted Chinese colleagues and friends who were able to care for me long enough and well enough to deliver me into Joan's waiting hands. I very much doubt I would have pulled through without that care. They attended to me constantly, now that I was a member of the hospital and medical school network, even helping to bathe and dress me. Their presence—the human concern, warmth, and support—sustained me and gave me hope, even when I had lost confidence in my body and, demoralized, almost gave up. I went to China to study trauma and its aftermath and ended up traumatized myself. My Chinese colleagues taught me that the moral responsibility to give care was more powerful and permanent than the sometimes transient circumstances of our lives. (And we experienced the reciprocity expected from such acts of care in real-world terms as we were called upon by these same colleagues over the decades to help them and their children come to the United States to train, study, and live.)

Joan led the way in our relationships with our many Chinese

students, colleagues, and friends. They valued her for the moral and emotional depth of her relationships with them—*renqing guanxi*. I led our academic collaborations, but Joan nurtured relationships of care and love. One of our earliest postdoctoral fellows was a young Hunanese psychiatrist who got into a bad accident— he was hit by a car while riding his bike in Boston—that damaged a knee and gave him a large lump on his forehead. My initial response was to scold him for having lied to us that he had health insurance, when in fact he had failed to purchase it in order to save the money and send it back to his family. Joan gently nursed him until he was able to walk. He never forgot what she did and the genuine warmth with which she did it. While I was tempted to criticize other Chinese research fellows for not putting enough effort into their research or writing, Joan always supported them, often working with them on remedial English-language and research skills. She took their responsibilities as her own, without complaining.

For Joan, classical Chinese poems and paintings offered occasions to make Chinese guests gain face and for her to share her broad knowledge of their cultural heritage. She also mastered the indirectness with which Chinese often convey emotions through metaphors of nature and the body, and she used these to support our friends in such a way as to neither embarrass them nor shock their sensibility. Handshakes were replaced with a bowing of the head; direct expressions of affection with a poetic phrase, a sad farewell with tears, not words. Thus, on June 4, 1989, as the Tiananmen Square massacre held a visiting Chinese researcher's eyes fixed on the TV with tears streaming down her face and inhaling huge gulps of air, Joan sat down beside her and held her hand, saying nothing but showing everything, later taking her back to our home to calm her agitation by massaging her back, feeling her pulse, feeding her cakes and tea, and sitting in our garden talking about plants and trees and the changing patterns of clouds.

I can remember several of our Chinese guests choking with sobs as they recounted the horrors they had experienced during the Cultural Revolution and the other radical Maoist political campaigns that went before it. Joan sat beside them holding their hands, her eyes moist with her own tears. She made herself fully present for them: warm, supportive, alive to what mattered to them. People would come to me about academic issues, but they sought out Joan to talk about personal problems and to enlist her advocacy and action on their behalf. But much of the time they (like me) just wanted to sit with her and soak up the love that washed over them in the form of care.

We were among the first Americans in the second half of the twentieth century to do research in China, starting only six years after Nixon's first visit there. In China, I returned to many of the same research questions that I had begun to explore in Taiwan, but I now added a new dimension. I wanted very much to understand the impact of the Cultural Revolution and other political campaigns on people's lives. What were their human costs? Had that trauma produced depression and anxiety disorders? Had it created biological symptoms and diseases? Could we determine the extent to which physical and psychological health had suffered in the wake of institutionalized brutality and mass shaming? We were able to study the psychological effects of these seismic upheavals—hunger and starvation, the imprisonments and torture, the forced displacements and relocations, the public shaming, the executions—on the Chinese population. Because we were doing medical research on depression, we could legitimately interview, without political interference, ordinary Chinese workers, cadres, intellectuals, and peasants who had been deeply injured by these devastating historical traumas.

Everything we had learned about the importance of family and friendship relationships was turned upside down by these destructive campaigns. During the worst of times, friend had turned on friend, family member had attacked family member. We studied the fragile efforts at repair and the bitter reality that the connections that were being remade carried the poison of past betrayals. No wonder that in the 1980s in China, on sidewalks and street corners, in markets and waiting rooms, in public parks or at dinner parties, people, usually apparent strangers, would occasionally explode in anger in response to a minor issue. Generations' worth of hate and hostility bubbled just below the surface.

During interviews with depressed patients, I encountered story after story of terrible injuries inflicted on people who came from "bad" class backgrounds, had "overseas problems" with family in Taiwan or the United States, had been "sent down" to remote, deeply impoverished rural areas, or had experienced the breakup of the family with members scattered all over China. Among these, the ones that stood out were those that represented harrowing injustices that had never been righted or even acknowledged as such. One young man as a schoolboy discovered a big-character poster (a damning and public political criticism) in the schoolyard that said "Down with Chairman Mao." The local authorities unfairly blamed him for writing it, and he was expelled from school, beaten, and sent to the distant countryside, where his anger mushroomed into a great hatred as he realized he would never be educated or have a fair chance in life.

It follows that in the current era of China's unprecedented

rise, families never talk about these earlier times. Grandchildren are kept largely ignorant. These traumas are not revisited, yet. The past is still too alive with bitterness (in its worst form, *qiside*, hatred unto death) and with regret to be safely explored without opening wounds that perhaps can never heal. So surprisingly, it is the outsider who can be entrusted with the dangerous words that would bend and break the relationships among insiders. People shared stories with us about a schoolchild who informed on his parents, sending each of them into distant exile for much of a decade; about a wife who beat her husband, blinding him in one eye and breaking and disfiguring his nose as part of a crowd that demanded his death; and about a weak and untrustworthy "friend," who repeatedly destroyed a colleague's career, family life, and personal health and happiness. Yet in most of these cases the family and relationships endured in some semblance of friendship, many even accommodating and surviving the occasional outburst of fury. The lesson for Joan and me was both tragic and sobering— sometimes even uplifting. People endure not only as broken individuals but also as part of networks that are scarred forever. The pain of misplaced loyalty, of past betrayal, of revenge, of resentment, and of unappeased hatred underlies the laughter, the happiness, and even the love they experience. American ideas of resilience, closure, and wholeness seem trite and immature when applied to these unspeakable conditions. Joan and I came to believe that the Chinese reality provided a deeper and more revealing account of how life is actually lived everywhere, because in a different if less destructive way, we, too, cannot escape the dire consequences of our divided history. I mean here that virtually every society has its own tortured history of oppression, suppression, violence, and usurpation that somehow must be overcome so ensuing generations can go on living. In the United States so much of this turns on race, class, political affiliation, gender, and for Jews especially, the Holocaust; in South Africa, it is about apartheid and goes beyond what the Truth and Reconciliation Commission's hearings tried to accomplish; in Rwanda it is ethnic genocide.

We learned that care can be given with presence and love in spite of hatred. But also that care can be refused in a relationship that superficially seems loving. Almost anything, it seemed to us at the time, could be endured, until it could not be endured for another moment.

Lee Xingwei helped bathe and feed her elderly husband, and did it with love, despite loathing him for being responsible for her parents' deaths during the Cultural Revolution. Qin Ruoyi lived together with her older sister, who suffered dementia, and took remarkable care of her, even though she could never forgive her for informing on her husband and thereby sending him to an early death in a labor camp. Our friend Nie Jinlin celebrated the ninetieth birthday of her father with toasts despite holding him responsible for her late mother's psychotic breakdown and years in a mental hospital because he publicly denounced her, then officially divorced her and married one of her enemies. To have maintained that relationship seems impossible, but for Nie, it was what she had to do to get through life. Think of the death camps of the Holocaust, as depicted by Primo Levi and others, where moral certainties were upended by the imperatives of survival. Or the moral ambiguities that lingered in post–World War II France over the question of collaboration with the Nazi occupiers. Or the members of communities who live with former enemies and torturers in their midst following periods of political chaos and persecution. Such morally gray areas persist even after the end of a war or a political movement. As a Chinese friend who lived through bad times concluded: "We are happy now. That is quite an achievement! We don't disturb these good times with bad thoughts. Why should we? But the past is not gone, nor forgotten. It lives within the present. It is carried by relationships, by individuals. That doesn't mean that it must be spoken or even valued. It is merely there. You get on with life."

As profoundly as my experiences in China altered my worldview, I am gratified that my work there also had a lasting effect on the Chinese. I had found that the leading diagnosis in Chinese clinics at the time, neurasthenia,* was a vague, catch-all classification. In Europe and the United States, most of those cases would have been described as depression and anxiety. In the early 1980s, even those cases that were treated with psychopharmacology and psychotherapy did not successfully resolve without addressing the family, workplace, or political issues they might involve. We were able to show that very often, patients' symptoms—their physical complaints—stood in for and symbolized political and social traumas. When we could confront those traumas, we could make progress in alleviating the physical and psychological symptoms.

China's senior psychiatrists did not take kindly to these findings, which they took to be a form of accusation that they were perhaps unable to diagnose depression or recognize its social sources. Their junior colleagues, however, being more in tune with global developments in the mental health field, took up the cause, and challenged how psychiatry was practiced in China.

---

* Neurasthenia was a term invented by an American neurologist in the 1860s, and globalized thereafter in Europe and later Asia. It was meant to convey the idea of the nervous system being overwhelmed by stress, leading to a breakdown of the nerves. The term was discarded in the United States by the early twentieth century but had stayed popular in China.

Ironically, though, I did not feel that all these developments actually led to improved professional care for Chinese patients. The health care system there failed to empower physicians through better training, by allowing them more time with patients, or by shifting the emphasis to the quality of the relationships between doctors and patients. My research got swept up in the race to improve the efficiency of the health care system, but it never brought about significant improvement in the quality of professional caregiving. Sadly, much the same could be said about the United States, where this kind of research is pretty well known, but not well aligned with the corporate interests and bureaucratic institutions that control health care.

Somehow the Chinese are getting on with life today. They can enjoy themselves in public. They can go out for dinner or to the movies, take vacation trips, watch TV programs, play recreational sports, knowing that as recently as the 1980s, no one could afford such things, even if they had been allowed. In those years, ordinary Chinese could not enter the big hotels or fancy restaurants, which were reserved for foreigners and the Chinese political elite.

The simple pursuit of everyday happiness is a relatively recent concept in China, as are quests of a more spiritual nature. Religions were attacked and at times prohibited under Mao, but many Chinese today are turning to Buddhism, Taoism, Christianity, Islam, and local folk practices for meaning and support. The rekindled interest in religion has triggered a new engagement with caregiving, in the community and at home. In the midst of dizzying economic changes and enhanced political repression of dissenters, where cynicism has flourished and personal values are often suspect, caregiving may well be the only truly liberating activity. Individuals and families can commit to caregiving practices that carry moral weight. The Chinese Communist state recognized the crucial value of care to China's traditions, its present concerns, and its future needs. The nation's leaders worry about a future, as a consequence of the one-child policy, in which there will be too few family members and workers to care for a greatly increased number of elderly. Here individual aspiration to care for a loved one and the social legitimacy of family caregiving as a way to maintain an otherwise fragile social security system reinforce each other.

Many Chinese cultural practices of self-care and self-cultivation are meant to deepen the mind-body relationship as a means to promote health, prevent disease, care for people with chronic illness, and lessen the effects of the aging process. The spectrum of bodily disciplines—from tai chi and *qigong* to martial arts, tonics, special diets, and nurturing the aging body-mind (*yang shen, yang lao*) through dance, singing, exercise, and pilgrimage—are part of a grand Chinese cultural health tradition of self-care and family care that connects ordinary people and the state, traditional Chinese medicine and modern public health. Joan taught me to respect and to learn from this vital cultural movement and also to recognize it as a sort of social care that embraces and connects Chinese individuals and the population as a whole. We can recognize cultural practices and movements in the United States too, which even though highly commercialized and remade by fads, signify a society-wide force of popular care. Think of the current craze in healthy diets (vegan, gluten-free, and pescatarian), exercise, and stress reduction through mindfulness and wellness (ironically, a secularized Asian import). The traditions are very different, and take on the cultural coloring of the places they are practiced, but in our globalized world the Asian and Western versions of these pursuits overlap and reinforce each other. It is not just the global political economy that is at work here; global culture is being built out of local traditions responding to existential life. That in turn has local consequences that develop differently.

Once again, we first perceive superficial cultural differences, which then give way to deeper existential similarities, which in turn disclose deep differences, finally revealing that there are but a limited number of ways of being human, but multiple versions of that universal humanity. Some are shared; some are not. We may argue about what human nature is and never come to agreement, but we can all recognize and acknowledge human conditions such as pain, suffering, joy, and care.

During this half century of ever-greater involvement with China and its people, I have learned that while I will always be an outsider, living in and with Chinese culture has enhanced both my social awareness to the world around me and my sensitivity to my own individuality. Joan knew this too. It is as if by cultivating Chinese relationships and meanings, we developed a sharper perspective on our own world and our own lives. Through this process, we also made ourselves more present to each other. We learned to care about, and for, the values and practices that had come to be central to our lives by participating in how others lived, and how they cared for what mattered to them. Our family grew stronger, our ties to each other tightened, and we advanced in our world as if we were cocooned from its pressures and dangers. But of course this was an illusion. Fate had other things in store for us.

Just before we left Taipei in 1979 after we concluded what would be our final research project there, Joan and I visited a famous fortune-teller. He was an old man, half asleep in the midday heat and drenching humidity in the corner of a large temple.

We performed the ritual and selected a fortune paper for him to interpret. He shook his head to fully waken himself and put on his eyeglasses to read the paper. He looked at it, then at each of us, and shook his head. We asked him what the fortune meant. Again he shook his head, and this time without speaking he waved us away. Joan, who had learned to read palms in college from a Rom student, whispered to me, "It must not be a good one. Once when I saw a bad sign on the palm of a friend, I refused to interpret it for her." The old man looked at us without smiling, pointed to the pile of fortune papers, and said softly, "Pick another!" Going forward, this was an unwelcome sign.

I recall the words of a Chinese patient whose depression I had treated successfully and whom I had gotten to know well. Addressing me by my Chinese name, he said: "Dr. Kai, you don't belong to our culture, but you know lots about it. And I can see how it has influenced you. What is not visible to you is how your culture has made you. But maybe by now both cultures have made you, gotten you ready to help me and others. Maybe, Dr. Kai, someday they will help *you* too."

Five

When I was in medical school, my early contact with patients—real human beings, each with their own unique human condition—lit a fire in me. Moving from basic science study in a classroom to practical, hands-on engagement with care gave the work the meaning that I hadn't even realized I was missing. As much as that care energized me, it is also in my nature to explore the intellectual underpinnings of the work we do, to seek order and patterns that become knowledge we can pass along to others. I am a practitioner, but I am also an academic, a researcher, a theorist. For a time, upon our return in 1970 from that first sojourn in Taiwan, I needed to nurture the more cerebral elements of my being and to shore up the theoretical foundations of my cross-cultural interests. I believed, and still do a half century later, that the human experiences of illness and healing need to be understood at their existential core through the human sciences in order to generate the deep knowledge that can improve caregiving and elevate its importance. Driven by this conviction, I went to Harvard, stepping away from the usual postgraduate clinical training track to immerse myself in a comparative study of medical systems across cultures.

It was an electrifying time, the air everywhere infused with social, political, and intellectual revolution. We arrived in Cambridge on a late summer afternoon to find hundreds of helmeted police in riot gear lined up in Harvard Square, grimly facing down a surging crowd of student protesters. After two years in Asia, we weren't used to civil unrest, but we would understand very quickly how so many of the customs, values, and behavior we had long taken for granted—loyalty to institutions and deference to authority, class and racial distinctions and hierarchies, the lockstep march through study, work, career, marriage, and family—had all been cast into doubt.

The early 1970s were also heady times for intellectuals and academics, as radically new schools of thought and analytical methodologies suddenly came into vogue. In a few short weeks, I realized that I could engage most deeply with all this important intellectual activity through anthropology. I fell in love with the field. Ethnography, the social study of the culture and lived practices of societies through deep immersion in fieldwork, resonated especially strongly with me. At that time, social and cultural anthropology, like other academic disciplines, was swept up in the cultural revolution that was roiling through the United States and Western Europe, and in the antiwar and civil rights movements that served as the moral fulcrum of that revolution. And yet, all the intellectual excitement came from breakthroughs in understanding the deep social structure and hidden cultural processes in small-scale preliterate societies in the highlands of Papua New Guinea, central and northern Australia, and the African and Latin American rainforests. Structural analyses and studies of symbol systems suggested universal ways in which human beings were connected to society. We learned how rituals created social memory, and legal, religious, economic, and even sexual relationships were organized as cultural systems. It was heady stuff that attracted philosophers, linguists, historians of science and religion, ethnomusicologists, and intellectuals in general. It meant that for a period of time social and cultural anthropology was at the very center of highly promising and broadly exciting interdisciplinary studies of human development.

I was hooked, particularly enamored of the symbolic anthropology advocated by Clifford Geertz at the University of Chicago. This approach emphasized the role of meaning in people's lives, meaning that became organized by a culture into systems that connected images and ideas with emotions and values. This way of thinking suggested that the world is physically real and tangible but at the same time is defined, categorized, and regulated by a cultural web that ensnares politics and economics. Cultural systems integrate meanings, feelings, and behaviors into local worlds that influence how we experience and express the body, how we construct social relationships, and how we evaluate moral and social goods. I appropriated this idea from symbolic studies and applied it to health and medicine, recognizing that these moral worlds define what matters most to people in the context of ill health, whether in a doctor's office, a research lab, or a patient's home.

Naturally, Joan and I came into contact with many new and truly interesting people in these exciting times. Among them would be one of the most influential figures in my life, the great champion of social medicine and pioneering child psychiatrist Leon Eisenberg. Leon was professor of psychiatry and one of the dominant Harvard intellectuals of the time. Beyond the realm of medicine, he advocated also for social justice and human rights, and together with his elegant Argentinian wife, Carola, also a psychiatrist—who was dean of students at MIT and would later be a dean at Harvard Medical School—formed the nucleus of one of the most fascinating networks in that rarefied world. Just a couple of weeks after we got to Cambridge, we found ourselves at a cocktail party at the Eisenbergs' house, a lively affair filled with laughter and conversation. There was Leon, in his shirtsleeves, surrounded by a rapt circle of listeners, waving a glass of beer as he held forth in a voice that everyone could hear above the thrum of the party. I wandered over, and was completely enchanted by the talk and its source. In a sense, I never left that spirited circle.

Of the many mentors and paternal figures in my life, Leon had the most far-reaching impact. A polymath of fearless and insatiable curiosity, he had amassed a storehouse of knowledge as vast as it was finely detailed. He had the wit and the verbal and mental agility to marshal all that information and send it into all sorts of battles, engaging his colleagues and friends in debates on any and all subjects. I recall traveling as his "junior" to a conference in Germany in 1972 called Creativity in Science, sponsored by a pharmaceutical firm and attended by such scientists and Nobel laureates as Jacques Monod and Nikolaas Tinbergen. Tinbergen, the world's leading ethologist (ethology is the study of animal behavior), conversed with Leon about the behavior of stippled trout and its implication for humans. When Leon excused himself to go to the bathroom, Tinbergen turned to me in amazement and wondered how it was that he had never come across the name of such a well-informed ethologist as Leon. He was even more impressed when I explained that Leon was a psychiatrist, not an ethologist. But it was a memorable meeting for more reasons than this. Monod and Leon, a Jew, approached our German host, the elderly CEO of the drug company, and inquired what the company had produced during the Nazi era. The CEO paled and looked as if he might faint. In fact, the company had manufactured the Zyklon B gas used in the death camps, knowledge of

which threw an entirely different and darker light on the festivi-
ties. I can't say if Leon knew this in advance, but it was a defining
characteristic of his persona to puncture superficial bubbles to
reveal darker truths.

Leon had associated himself with the political Left in the
1940s and '50s, and as a result, his name appeared on many of the
notorious blacklists of the era. He maintained that politics determined all economic conditions. His social approach to medicine
reflected the socialist values behind the work of many of the most
seminal figures in our field, all of whom influenced my thinking
and my work. One of these was Rudolf Virchow, a German physician and anthropologist of the nineteenth century who approached medicine as a social science and put forth the idea that
poverty and other social conditions are determining factors in
health and disease. To my mind, that made social suffering the
basis of medicine. I was also greatly inspired by W. H. R. Rivers,
who worked as both a psychiatrist and an anthropologist. The
method of psychiatry that I would develop incorporated aspects
of the ethnographic approach that Rivers pioneered in the South
Pacific and then employed to treat military officers traumatized
by World War I. The psychiatrist enters the local world of the
patient figuratively just as an anthropologist enters as a professional stranger—a "marginal native"—into the real local world of
another society. Once there, the therapist's job is to help the patient face up to what is most threatening in the illness experience
and most at stake in the treatment.

Globally, from Europe to Latin America and elsewhere, researchers and theorists were working at the intersection of medicine and social science, reevaluating the delivery of health care in
the context of broader social conditions. In South Africa, physicians like Sidney Kark, John Cassel, and Mervyn Susser were

working with leaders of the anti-apartheid movement to build community clinics in underserved areas, providing cost-effective care and prevention in the face of crushing economic and social disparity. They were brave champions of social justice and public health, who were driven out of South Africa by the government but carried on their work—which included pioneering the field of social epidemiology—around the world. That research method became part of the field of social medicine, which Leon and others would revive at Harvard. It became my intellectual home.

Leon Eisenberg's influence tempered my infatuation with the subtleties of social structures and cultural symbol systems that were all the rage in academic circles. He helped me see how those systems were conditioned by the brute force of colonialism, imperialism, and behind it all, the varieties of voracious capitalism. The primary agenda for me, my generation of medical anthropologists, and our students would be how, in our analyses, to balance political economics and sociocultural processes as they affected in particular the physical, psychological, and emotional lives of poor and marginalized people. Leon made clear that our subject would have to be broad enough to range from social suffering, through the lives of ordinary people and professionals, to social revolution or, at the very least, social change. Unlike public health, it would elevate care to the same stature as prevention. In other words, the goal was not to prevent disease but care for those who were already suffering. Indeed, care would become the path to prevention, as my own students Paul Farmer and Jim Kim would demonstrate decades later for AIDS and tuberculosis.

Leon considered everything relevant; nothing was inconsequential. The more awareness and knowledge one carried, the deeper the meaning and resonance of every interaction. Passionately committed to excellence in academic and clinical work, he had carried out the first controlled clinical trial in child psychiatry and immersed himself in anything and everything that piqued his intellectual curiosity. Leon's fiercest commitment was to social justice and human rights. He represented everything I aspired to become—a critically minded scholar, hands-on researcher, social revolutionary thinker, and wise clinician. He was teacher, role model, father confessor, cheerleader, carer, and more. I don't know if I would have fashioned the career I have had without him.

I learned from him to take everything in and to filter, organize, and synthesize it through all that I had experienced, studied, or debated, to arrive at an understanding of what could best help real people and improve society. From the smallest details to the biggest ideas, he taught me how to apply critical inquiry to things medical and social, and to link them in a great chain of rethinking and reform. Not least, he demonstrated that theory could and, in fact, must guide practical experience. He recognized my inveterate faults, and like Joan modeled a different and better way of being in the world. He also taught me how to laugh at pretense, my own included, and how to carry myself as a man: seriously but lightly, full of ideals but treading firmly on the ground. (In my lectures, even today, I still tell some of Leon's best jokes to lighten the more sobering lessons!)

In those first years at Harvard, I took my MA in anthropology and basically trained myself to create a new kind of medical anthropology focused on clinical relevance. I also completed my residency in psychiatry under Leon at the Massachusetts General Hospital. Here, too, the radical iconoclastic spirit of the times, which encouraged men and women of all fields to question established wisdom, nudged me to develop a new concept of cultural psychiatry. My approach upended the dominant psychiatric knowledge, which was based primarily on studies of white subjects, who accounted for only 20 percent of the globe's population, and which was minimally nuanced by data from the other 80 percent of people of color in the world. Seen that way, psychiatry had to change its priorities and practices to ones more in keeping with what is known today as global mental health. I pursued research in the United States and Taiwan as a postdoctoral fellow on cultural influences on depression and how people with mental health problems were failed by the health care system.

I practiced psychotherapy too. The very first therapy patient I had was well known to the hospital as a disruptive woman in her midtwenties who had been diagnosed with borderline personality disorder, meaning that she lived right at the border between psychosis and neurosis, which she could cross for minutes, hours, or longer periods of time. I recall meeting her at the door of a small therapy room that had two chairs separated by a table with a vase, and an internal window opening onto one of the hospital's busy walkways. I introduced myself, but she responded with only an odd and intense gaze. We sat in silence for perhaps thirty seconds, and then in a blinding motion she grabbed the vase and hurled it through the internal window, shattering the glass and the vase and startling the staff and patients on the walkway.

She glared at me defiantly and snarled, "You are the worst psychiatrist I have ever met."

I responded with a calmness that surprised me and belied how angry I felt. "That may well be. But you couldn't possibly know that in the minute we have spent together!" I paused then to reassure hospital security that I could handle her, which I wasn't really sure was true, and with all the authority I could muster, told her, "I will continue to see you, but you must never do anything like that again. I won't reject you, if that is what you fear, and thus feel you need to reject me first. But first we need to settle on a ground rule—nothing like this again. OK?"

"OK," she replied, and we went on to see each other through three years of weekly therapy, during which time she appeared in the psychiatry emergency room much less frequently than in the past, or in the years to come after I left Boston. This patient never became easy. She periodically became psychotic, and she shared hair-raising stories, such as when she got so angry at a dinner companion that she set the tablecloth on fire, or how she was sure the silverware was threatening her whenever she turned her back. I learned the importance of acknowledging her experience without judgment or criticism, allowing my empathy to affirm her personhood, no matter how difficult she became. We focused on the things that helped her struggle with her cruel disorder, but the real revelation was that the process we went through together made it possible for me to endure her intractable behavior as well. The experience helped reveal to me the reciprocal nature of care.

Patients like this woman taught me a key value: In spite of how challenging or painful a patient might be for the professional, the patient's suffering counts more than your suffering. You can sit with people in the deepest pain—whether it's the physical pain endured by the little girl covered with burns, or the psychic pain suffered by this woman with borderline personality disorder— and be with them in their terrible experience, so that your very presence in and of itself can be a powerful source of care. While their wounded and needy presence provides the raison d'être for keeping the relationship going, you must recognize and master your own needs and wounds. You can, and must, control your anger and frustration and, no matter how confrontational the situation, withstand the pressure the patient's behavior inflicts on you. You will yourself to absorb the hostility and hate. But it is the reciprocal relationship that matters most in caregiving. So these responses need to be understood as efforts to keep the relationship going.

I had in mind, as well, a most memorable patient from those early days of psychotherapy who was a brilliant researcher and who, as I described in *The Illness Narratives*, had produced a fictitious disease by injecting himself with an anticlotting factor antibody (which he had created in the laboratory) that produced a bleeding disorder that none of the specialists could figure out. This behavior was my entrée into the tragic story he told me of being scarred and abandoned by a psychotic mother and finding solace only in acts of self-harm that convinced him that he was really alive and receiving the punishment he felt he deserved. Totally alone and isolated, he counted as his only "friends" a pickled snake and a skeleton he kept in his home. Sitting with him and hearing out his bizarre tale of horror and desperate loneliness, I had to reach deep within my resources of compassion and imagination to put myself—without judgment or aversion—into the terrible reality he endured. While in therapy with me he stopped mutilating himself and manufacturing fictitious diseases. But like many patients with this kind of dangerous behavior, he eventually dropped out of treatment and I never heard from or about him again. This was a caregiving relationship that could not be maintained.

Because my clinical specialty was consultation-liaison psychiatry, in which I was called into a hospital setting in internal medicine and surgery to see patients who had delirium, psychosis, depression, or other psychological conditions, the vast majority of cases I saw were less memorable but equally formative for me. And yet I was taken with how these patients' stories shaped their symptoms and served to either hasten or block their treatment. For instance, I was called by an internal medicine resident to see a patient the doctor thought was psychotic because she was urinating frequently and vomiting without a clear-cut medical reason. I discovered—simply asking her about what she understood to be her problem and what she was doing about it—that she was a poorly educated daughter and wife of plumbers who held, not surprisingly, a plumber's view of her body: water coming in and water going out. Told that she had congestive heart failure and that there was "water" in her lungs, she was sensibly trying to rid her body of that water, in keeping with her understanding of how the body works.

Other patients felt overwhelmed by anxiety, paralyzed by depression, and hopeless and helpless in the face of grave medical conditions and frightening treatments. Their fears were often compounded by deeply personal problems having to do with work, family, or money. The residents and attending physicians took a detailed medical history but focused almost exclusively on the details of the patients' biomedical pathology and their pharmacological or surgical treatment. To my mind, it seemed equally important to patients' care to understand the details of their lives and to get them to verbalize their perspective on their own illness. I constructed a clinical and research methodology out of this vast field of experiences, to which many clinicians seemed blind and deaf. I devised eight "explanatory model" questions intended to elicit the patient's and family's views of the cause, course, and treatment and what mattered most to them about their problems. At first, I was delighted to see this methodology widely read and taught, but I later became frustrated to realize it had simply become just another element of the routine examination checklist, curtailed also perhaps by the unremitting pace and time demands of medical consultations, and not the conversation starter I had intended—a tool for connecting physicians and patients on a more fundamental human level. I envisioned the clinician as an ethnographer of the worlds of patients and their social networks and believed that we could bring anthropology and social science more generally to bear on clinical work. That is exactly how Anne Fadiman used my approach in her influential book, *The Spirit Catches You and You Fall Down,* to point to a better way to treat patients and families from the Hmong community in California.

Let's imagine that you are a doctor or nurse presented with an adolescent girl with poorly controlled diabetes. You figured out that she was not complying with the diet or the insulin regimen. But why was that? If you stopped at identifying the problem, rather than digging into the cause of her behavior, you would have disempowered yourself as a therapist and probably lost the chance to change behavior that could have profoundly negative consequences for her health. Why not find out about how her self-image, relationships with family and friends, experiences in school and after-school activities, and personal aspirations and fears all influenced her decisions not to follow the onerous diet or her unwillingness to be constrained by a medical regimen for life? Probing those social and personal and even hormonal influences (after all, she is a teenager) can make all the difference in breaking her destructive pattern of self-care. Yes, it takes time, real interest, and commitment to understand these factors, but if coming to terms with them can yield positive change, it simply has to happen. Multiply such cases by the tens or hundreds of thousands and you completely upend the cost-effectiveness equation that health economists and policy makers rely on these days.

My thinking about care continued to evolve. From the Yale clinical epidemiologist Alvan Feinstein, I had adopted but refined the distinction between *illness* (the patient's experience of symptoms and functional limitation) and *disease* (the disordered biomedical processes affecting the body). In my formulation, *illness* stood for the way patients and families first encountered, processed, and responded to symptoms, while *disease* was the result of any practitioner's (biomedical professional, chiropractor, traditional Chinese medicine practitioner, folk healer) understanding of the cause and nature and outcome of the pathology. This was a rare case where I parted ways with Leon, for whom biomedicine was part of an almost sacrosanct realm of science, and therefore on a higher plane than other healing systems not based on science. Influenced by the work of Thomas Kuhn, author of the groundbreaking *The Structure of Scientific Revolutions*, for whom all science was a human project, of Bruno Latour, who carried out an ethnography of a biomedical research lab as if it were a native village, and others, I insisted that even what we held to be objective scientific reality had to be examined as socially constructed truth.

Over time, this illness/disease distinction seemed to me less and less tenable. After all, patients were increasingly aware of, and using, biomedical and other healing systems' views of pathology to identify and treat their health problems. Feeling newly empowered, and with access to so much more information, patients and their families added their own perceptions and ideas about illness and health to those promulgated by governments and businesses. And, of course, our basic scientific understanding was constantly evolving. After all, I had been taught in medical school that diabetes was caused by an insufficiency of insulin. But once researchers showed that insulin receptors could be disordered so that there was too much insulin in some cases of diabetes, we had to reconsider that long-established idea.

And so there was an ongoing interplay of biological science, social science, and political economic processes that rendered many of the simple distinctions I had introduced to improve clinical practice no longer intellectually tenable or clinically useful. It was as if in each historical period, a new conceptual framework needed to be introduced to keep professional practitioners focused on the patients' experience of illness and treatment, while the patient and family needed to come to a more sophisticated understanding of what was problematic in care so that they could make more appropriate demands and advocate more effectively for reform. The ultimate goal for patients—perhaps not completely shared by medical educators, policy makers, and designers of health care systems—was to make medicine more attentive to their needs, as well as to their lives more broadly.

My experiences in the clinic and hospital repeatedly disturbed my view of how medicine should be practiced. Late one afternoon I was called by a neurosurgery resident, who implored me to come quickly to the surgical waiting room and to tell the family that the patient had died on the operating table. Shocked, I told him I didn't know his patient or the family, but I did know it was his moral responsibility to speak to the family members about this devastating event and explain fully how it happened. "You're the psychiatrist, you know how to speak to people," he begged. "OK," I responded, "I will help you and we will do it together. But understand, I will be there to stand beside you. It is your responsibility to face up to this sad situation and to sit with them and bear the pain with them. It is going to be tough but you must do this and you will."

Admittedly, and fortunately, this only happened once in my experience, yet it powerfully illustrates my building sense that something was terribly wrong with how physicians, and especially high-technology-oriented specialists, practiced. It was as if I could see *care* disappearing before my very eyes. On another occasion I was going through tape recordings from doctor-patient interactions in a primary care setting. A physician was working with an untrained interpreter who was the family member of an elderly patient who had been acting worried at home. The physician prompted the family member to ask if the patient was hearing voices. He did this to determine if she was psychotic and hallucinating. "Yeah," said the patient in Chinese, "I can hear your voice and the doctor's." Her family member replied to the doctor in English, "Yes she is hearing voices, she says." The outcome of what otherwise would be comic was the truly dangerous mistake of giving a prescription for a powerful antipsychotic medication with strong and potentially dangerous side effects to a patient who was not psychotic but, as it later turned out, was in part actively worried about her financial situation. I could understand the Chinese-English translation confusion, and I corrected this medical error and prevented a potentially serious complication, but I still couldn't understand how the physician failed to use a trained medical interpreter or to explain to the unwitting family member that he (the physician) was trying to determine if the patient had hallucinations, and not a hearing problem.

So many of the patients I was asked to evaluate complained that either nothing had been explained to them about their illness and treatment, or so little that they couldn't understand what was happening. It seemed as if medicine was being practiced in a veterinary mode. I said this in a radio interview and was roundly (and appropriately) criticized by a veterinarian who explained that vets often know their animals well and explain in detail to the owners about what the problem is and how it should be treated. I may have used the wrong analogy, but the point still holds. The serious problem in patient-doctor communication is nothing new; it has been decades in the making. I venture that it has worsened in recent years, as increasingly complicated electronic technologies come between doctors and patients, with the machines' ever-present demands to be fed data further eating into the practitioners' time and inclination to inquire into their patients' lives and concerns. The sheer pace of medical rounds and procedures in hospital wards often leaves no time for engaging patients or family members as fellow travelers in their treatment and recovery. This can be devastating for junior doctors whose expectations for quality care are dashed by the unforgiving and unrelenting world of underresourced and overpressured hospital medicine. I am reminded of one young resident who had talked enthusiastically of becoming a geriatric specialist, who—at the end of yet another long and harrowing day of barked orders with no respite, even to eat, or supervisory support—sobbed with exhaustion, anger, and despair, saying, "I used to love old people, but now I don't care." Perhaps it is dehumanizing experiences like this that not only harden the defensive shells of some doctors and nurses but contribute to anxiety, depression, and suicides.

Nor do many patients fare much better, particularly in public hospitals where the resources fall so far short of the need. Recently a report by the National Academy of Medicine showed that there is so little communication by surgeons and nurses about home-based aftercare for surgical patients that when patients return home confused and worried, after a night or two in the hospital following a surgical procedure, their family carers are at a total loss as to what to do with the drains emerging from the patients' bodies. Most have never been given an explanation of how to care for their family member at home. Could any silence be more damning than this one? Clearly, what was a serious problem when I was in medical school fifty years ago has risen to the level of a crisis in health care today. I have watched with escalating dismay and frustrated alarm as caregiving in medicine has gone from bad to worse.

In 1974, I published four articles in different medical and social science publications that more or less defined the next forty-plus years of my work on caregiving. One examined medicine as a cultural system and asked which issues that cultural lens clarified or obscured for practitioners. In other words, did the culture of medicine itself create these issues? Another article proposed a broader comparative model of health care in which family and network care, largely overlooked at that time by public health models, figured prominently, and professional and folk practices were seen from the layperson's perspective as vital components in a broader system of care. That system was defined neither by hospitals and clinics, nor by public health's professional logic, but rather by patient and family interests and the resources they sought out to act on those interests. (Tellingly, drug and medical device companies knew what public health experts didn't and were increasingly advertising directly to patients and families.)

In these papers I was coming to terms with the revelations that would shape my career. To begin with, the practice of medicine was only one example of the far broader practice of care. Second, care itself was based on what truly mattered in the illness and treatment experience for patients and practitioners. And what mattered differed for professional, personal, and social reasons. And third, this more patient-oriented approach applied not just to health care in Boston and the rest of the United States, but to what I had observed and studied in Taipei and, later still, Changsha. By including that cross-cultural comparison, the question of care became not only a professional and a layperson's issue but also a societal issue. I had come to see that illness and care were inseparable from what defined a society. Moreover, because I was able to examine radically different societies in my own work, and to explore through my reading so many other societies around the world, I could see that to some extent, this was true about the existential human condition everywhere. And I could also see at a very early stage the global changes in health care systems—the enormous growth of bureaucratic regulation, the flood of public and private capital, the loss of professional autonomy and proletarianization of practitioners, and the greatly expanded influence of Big Pharma and the health insurance companies—that were creating the problems that are now common worldwide.

Much of what I am writing may not seem so radical or revelatory to an informed person today, but five decades ago this was neither lay nor professional common sense. The field of care, and how we understand and practice it, has changed fundamentally. And I have been there both before and after that transformation.

In 1976, I was offered two jobs. First was an opportunity to remain at Harvard in an untenured assistant professorship at the Harvard School of Public Health that carried with it the chairmanship of a department of health and social behavior. The position would have kept me very much in the circle of mentors in which I was thriving. The other offer was for a tenured associate professorship in the Department of Psychiatry and Behavioral Sciences with an accompanying adjunct associate professorship in anthropology at the University of Washington in Seattle, a place to which we had hardly any connection and a city where we had never lived. As enticing as the Harvard job was, it did not include the opportunity for a deeper academic engagement with my new love, anthropology. It took about two minutes for Joan to make the fateful decision for our family. We would go to Seattle and the University of Washington for the tenure, which meant more stability and more control over our own lives. Although I could not have expressed it at the time, this, too, was an important kind of care, care for the family's future and for our individual development.

Six

Our arrival in Seattle marked the beginning of a long period of stability and calm for our family, and of high productivity for Joan and me. It really was the prime of our adult lives, but in fact, my first few days at work made me reconsider whether we had made the right choice. The chair of the Department of Psychiatry, who had recruited me, happened to join me in the elevator as I rode up to my new office. He asked me warmly if I was pleased by the tenure appointment, which he let me know he had fought hard to make happen. "Of course," I replied with a big smile, at which point he invited me into his office to talk about "other small matters."

Apparently, in the rush of recruitment, he had forgotten to mention a little something. It turned out that in addition to heading the Division of Social and Cultural Psychiatry, he also expected me to act as chief of the Consultation-Liaison Psychiatry Service, the doctors who are brought in by other medical specialists in the hospital wards when they believe a patient needs psychiatric evaluation or attention. This had constituted the bulk of my clinical work at Harvard. I blanched, my mind racing, desperately trying to work out how I could take on this large clinical responsibility while also handling a professorship in anthropology and spending each summer on my research in Taiwan, which I was scheduled and funded to do. More than all these considerations, I had books inside me I needed to get out.

"Look," he said, laughing lightly, "you'll get used to it. And it isn't nearly as big a deal as it sounds. Don't take our six hospitals too seriously—you have good attendings in each one. All you have to do is oversee the teaching and research and the quality of clinical service." The quality of clinical service at six hospitals! It sounded impossible. I couldn't imagine how I would pull it off.

In a state of extreme agitation, I went on to introduce myself to the half dozen residents assigned to my service who were congregating outside the chair's door. I was to be their leader, but I was only one year out of my own training. They walked me around, showing me the way to the internal medicine ward. The chief of gastroenterology, a world-renowned expert who four years later would treat me for an illness I acquired in China, walked up to our group and introduced himself.

Deadpan, he said, "I know you come from Mass General and Harvard where they believe this sort of thing but I think you should know that here we don't believe the mind has any effect on the gut!" I stood in amazement, wondering if I had actually heard him right. The mind having no effect on the gastrointestinal system was a ridiculous, totally insupportable idea. Decades of research and hundreds of research papers proved a powerful connection. I walked away shaking my head, thinking the guy was a barbarian, and wondering what I had gotten myself into. I later learned that unlike the chair of psychiatry, the chief had really been pulling my leg. Still reeling from the revelation of the unmanageable extent of my new responsibilities, I literally walked into the professor of transplant surgery, who would later on also become a friend. Jabbing at me with his index finger, he nearly shouted, "Kleinman, I have had so much trouble with psychiatry residents seeing my patients that I will only allow you yourself to see them."

I protested in a panic. "But this is a teaching hospital, and all transplant patients need to have psychiatric evaluation. I couldn't possibly see them all; even the residents will barely manage, given everything else they have to do."

"No, my friend, only you." And with that, he walked away.

Probably at this point I had most of the symptoms of mild clinical shock. I was without words, and only partly verbal throughout the rest of that day, which would go down as one of the worst days of my life. How could I possibly function in this place and do all the things on my academic agenda? That night, I asked Joan in all sincerity if she had unpacked everything, and when she said no, I suggested she hold off on that; so bad was my day that we might have to crawl back to Boston.

"Take it easy," she said, smiling, rubbing my shoulders and back. "Things will get better. Tomorrow is your anthropology day!"

And so it was. I arrived at the department office the next day and asked the administrator how to get to the seminar room that was assigned for the course I was to be teaching that day. "Oh no!" she said, laughing. "You're not in a seminar room. In fact, you're not in our lecture hall either. You're in the large lecture hall across the way." Another day, another jolt. I had been under the impression that I would be teaching an introductory seminar on medical anthropology with thirty or so students, much like the course I had established at Harvard. I have never taught a lecture course, I remember thinking as I opened the door to a lecture hall filled with over four hundred students. I must have looked like I was about to flee, because one of the graduate student teaching fellows caught my arm and introduced me to her five or six colleagues, who seemed to be cowering in a corner. "We had to turn students away," she said softly. "There are lots more who said that they wanted to take the course."

Somehow I survived the lecture and day two, and then the first few crazy weeks that followed. I was no stranger to hard work, but this enormous load was pushing me to a much higher level. Slowly I got used to the overburdened schedule and frenetic pace. And over time, once I found my sea legs, I flourished, much as Joan said she knew I would, in a setting in which I could build my own programs and projects and do the work exactly as I saw fit.

While Joan did graduate work in Chinese language and literature and managed our family affairs, my six years in Seattle saw my career and reputation blossom. I pursued the research projects in Taiwan that formed the basis of my first book, *Patients and Healers in the Context of Culture* (1980). The book became a founding text in medical anthropology, and earlier still I launched a new journal called *Culture, Medicine, and Psychiatry* (1977), which is still thriving, and an accompanying book series, which no longer exists. I threw myself into teaching at all levels: undergraduates, graduate students, medical students, and residents. And I did a huge amount of clinical work, seeing hundreds of patients—some in a pain clinic to which I consulted, others in the medical and surgical wards, and a number in my private practice. Looking back, I can scarcely believe I did even half these things. The deep dive into clinical work was the best thing that could have happened to me. As the years passed, I began to make connections between people's symptoms, their social lives, and what they believed was at risk for them and their loved ones on an existential level. I worked out new ideas about how culture patterned what people complained about and the way they complained; how each illness experience took a particular social course; how patients' life stories had unique themes and motifs that one could identify, beyond the commotion of complaints and the testimonies of distress. And that with intense listening and a psychotherapist's sensibility to the inner life, one could hear the subtle swelling or diminishing tone behind the spoken words. Those rising and falling notes connected with demoralization and depression that could be addressed directly. Ideally, such carefully focused treatment could break cycles of dangerous and destructive illness behavior, such as patients not adhering to the medical regimen, or exaggerating complaints to get the attention they needed, or conversely, denying the seriousness of their problems and the need for treatment. Moreover, I learned how to demonstrate these clinical approaches to students so that clinical rounds with postdoctoral fellows and other trainees became small performances. Nowhere was this more apparent than with chronic pain patients in the University of Washington's multidisciplinary pain clinic.

Jennifer Williams was a single, middle-aged accountant who for over two years had experienced disabling lower back pain that brought her to this nationally recognized clinic. Neither her primary care physician nor three orthopedic and neurosurgical consultants had been able to determine what was causing the pain. The imaging examinations revealed no significant pathology, nor did other tests. She was placed in the category of unexplained symptoms/chronic pain. Her family and friends had given up on her and were suspicious that the pain was not "real." She felt stigmatized as a "chronic complainer." The company that had employed her had finally run out of patience, and Jennifer was negotiating with it and with the disability system for workers' compensation so that she would not have to return to work, which she claimed made the pain worse. She had also gotten into a tense relationship with her primary care doctor over her requests for opioid pain relievers. Jennifer had all the symptoms of depressive disorder with the added hazard of addiction to medications.

She told me that because no one believed her about how serious her pain was, she had come to feel hopeless and helpless. When I told her I believed her, she seemed surprised, and the trainees gathered around me were clearly startled. I explained that I meant I believed she was experiencing serious pain in her back. Obviously, the doctors remained uncertain about the cause of her pain and therefore remained suspicious about her disability. But that she was suffering greatly from the pain, I had no doubt. Then I had a long talk with her. She told me things that no one on the medical team had heard. Jen, as she liked to be called, lived alone and had no close friends. Casting her eyes down toward the floor, her face reddened, she sobbed as she told me that obesity had been a problem since childhood. She had experienced shaming and bullying on account of it. Worse yet, she had been physically and sexually assaulted by older students. This web of dreadful events had led her to make a suicide attempt, after which she underwent a brief involuntary psychiatric hospitalization. Following that, she accused her family of failing to support her and ran away from home. She still felt relatively distant from her family. She clutched my hand as she kept repeating: "I am a failure. I can't control anything in my life. The pain isn't just in my back. It's in my head, beating me down."

The trainees almost gasped when I told Jen she had been heroic in the face of such overwhelming distress. "You have done all you could in the face of so much adversity. You have been extraordinarily brave. Now let us help." I implored, "Let us get the right treatments going for your depression and your pain. Who wouldn't be depressed by such pain—in your back but also as you say in your head and in your life."

Jen thanked me and told me I was the first doctor she had met who truly seemed to understand how her whole life was affected. After we left her and walked to a nearby conference room to discuss her case, the trainees expressed amazement that I had elicited in a few minutes a story that none of her other doctors had known about over the course of several years. "No magic here," I told them. "It's quite likely they never asked her in a way that made her feel they were on her side and truly interested in her, not just in the pain. When you are talking with chronic pain patients, you need to begin by realizing they have usually been caught up in terribly troubled relations where their pain is felt as a certainty by them but is doubted by doctors and family members, making for an impossible, nontherapeutic relationship of mutual distrust. Cut the Gordian knot—tell each patient you encounter that the pain is real, which it is, and that you believe them. [This assumes that actual malingerers are small in number, which they are.] You can also tell them that while the pain is real, it is still uncertain what is causing it, so you need to work on that too. In my experience, most of the time they will thank you and accept treatment for depression and for pressing personal and social problems. In turn, such treatment will often improve their mental state and social relationships and motivation to take on a therapeutic exercise regimen, and with it at the very least lessen the effect of the pain (which again, in my experience, is both on the body and on the psyche) enough to enable them to be more active and thereby reduce the disablement. At best, they will become fully functioning again. But most of the time they will continue to feel the pain but perceive it as less severe, thereby improving their lives at home and at work."

And indeed, when treated for her depression and the contrib-uting life problems with psychotherapy and an antidepressant medication, Jen improved enough to see a physical therapist, begin a weight-loss program with a dietitian, and work with an athletic trainer. Even after her depression lifted, she continued in psycho-therapy, working on issues of trauma, sexual abuse, and problems of self-image, sexual identity, and her greatly strained family rela-tions. The last time I heard from her, she was three years out from our earlier time together and had lost significant weight, improved her self-image, was actively practicing yoga, and had changed her job to work in a larger and more supportive firm that had rewarded her with a higher level of responsibility. She was also in a relation-ship with a woman whom she loved. Jen thanked me profusely and said something to this effect: "You alone believed me and believed in me. You understood how depressed I was at the time. I didn't tell you that I had suicidal thoughts, I lied on that one. But if I had gone on with that horrible situation much longer I might have tried to kill myself. I hope all those students with you will grow up to be a good doctor like you. Thank you."

I used this case to make the point to the students that the bu-reaucratization of health care had led to a serious loss of caring and caregiving among professionals. Physicians spent most of their time in such deadening bureaucratic tasks as filling out forms, searching through masses of test results, speaking on the phone with insurance company representatives, arguing with case managers over time available to talk with patients, and the like. They got paid for simple diagnoses and the straightforward treat-ments they implied. You, as a patient, either met the criteria for a billable condition or you didn't. We were losing nuance, ambigu-ity, complexity, and subtlety in assessing people and their real-life problems. If you focus only on someone's pain and consider that pain only from a disease perspective, you miss the context, the life of the sufferer, and with those essential signals, the opportunity to understand pain as communication and to participate in that communicative process in a way that can be clinically helpful and might even transform the relations that amplify the pain and thereby reduce its negative effects.

I went back to the idea of medicine as a bureaucracy. Max Weber, the German sociologist, reasoned that bureaucracies were concerned with *efficiency*, and efficiency required a simplified, even simplistic rationalization of human actions that removed all that was spontaneous, emotion-laden, morally important, and deep—in other words, all that was most human. What was happening to medicine in our time illustrated what Weber had theorized.

So these teaching rounds at the University of Washington, which I would later continue at Harvard Medical School and its affiliated hospitals (especially at the then Cambridge Hospital) for much of my academic career, enabled me to demonstrate interviewing skill—perhaps my only authentic research skill— along with teaching about anthropological, ethical, and global health perspectives on particular cases that helped resolve the clinical questions those cases raised. This teaching strategy also illustrated larger themes such as how race, ethnicity, gender, social class, poverty, and homelessness affected patients and practitioners and health care systems generally.

After the students had observed the interviews I was doing, my conversations with them encouraged their critically minded reflections on the problems at hand. These conversations were also constructed as academic colloquies in which they could discuss how history, social theory, and ethnography could be made directly pertinent to the clinic, and also the basis for a broader understanding of the social processes and structures affecting health care systems and the people who used them. Thus, Robert Merton's idea of the unintended consequences of social action was a useful way of understanding how a single one-size-fits-all intervention to control chronic pain, like a surgical procedure, could create side effects that worsened or prolonged the pain. (What was needed was a team approach that examined the interplay of all the relevant factors and also provided caring relationships, an approach this pain clinic had indeed pioneered and that later on would become routine in cancer care.) For Merton, an American sociologist, our "rigidity of habit" and "the imperious immediacy of interest"—both of which accurately describe medical personnel under pressure of doing something quickly to relieve a patient's pain—would invariably blind us to the unanticipated repercussions of our actions. So, for example, chronic pain would be treated only with a prescription for opioid pain medication. Imagine this insight applied to the United States as a whole, and add the financial motives of pharmaceutical companies, the pursuit of profit by a large part of the health sector, and the perilous position of those who cannot afford medical insurance, and we begin to understand at least one of the origins of the opioid crisis.

Similarly, Michel Foucault's idea of biopower—which proposes that medical treatment can be a means of governmental control—helped students think about the intended effects of policies that regulate pain medications, which brings the government into the process of clinical care, or the relationship between pain and disability, where the US disability system, which primarily affects people from the working class, is one of the limited means of income redistribution in our country. The medicalization of what in earlier eras were defined as social welfare problems, such as poverty and its effects on human lives, offers another example of how health care systems serve purposes that go far beyond medicine and represent how our society is regulated and governed. For students this is an opportunity to talk about the frustrating role of doctors as gatekeepers to societal resources and failed healers for forms of social suffering, like poverty, that their individual actions cannot resolve. Perhaps—armed with this appreciation of why their professional care is subverted by frustrating bureaucratic tasks that contribute to disillusionment—medical students and young doctors can defend themselves against burnout.

In the same way, introducing students to my idea about local moral worlds—the networks and organizations that we belong to where what is most valued by the group may be at odds with our personal inner sense of what is right—can prepare them for the reality of practice in a for-profit hospital where the emphasis on giving the highest-quality care often collides with the constraints of minimizing expenditures and satisfying the shareholders. Maybe those students will gain insight into how the ethos of a health policy office in which subjective patient complaints count less than quantitative measures of treatments can distort the meaning of quality of care. Or maybe they'll learn to see through the eyes of a patient how an emphasis on enhanced efficiency, which makes a clinic look good in the eyes of its administrators, can reduce the quality of care by removing the doctor from her core tasks of caregiving and insisting she spend more of her time with the computer screen or with health insurance representatives. I have found that this teaching strategy opens the eyes of students and practitioners to how their professional lives are shaped by large socioeconomic and political forces, and why, if they want to protect caregiving in health care systems, they need to take an active role in society's democratic institutions as concerned and informed citizens. Many of my students come away feeling that they must engage with community advocacy, policy making, and practical actions of resistance to the dominant social forces of our time, such as governmental laws undermining the care they give.

I began to include anthropology graduate students on these hospital rounds; we gave them the somewhat awkward name "clinically applied anthropology rounds." (One surprised pharmacist whose mother had been visited during these "anthropology rounds," laughed, and asked, "What do you think she is, a cave woman?") I was trying to integrate the ethnographic, social theory, diagnostic, and psychotherapeutic sides of my own hybrid world into an anthropological approach to clinical medicine, especially as it related to patients with chronic noncommunicable diseases like arthritis, asthma, diabetes, and chronic heart disease. For these patients, even a 10 percent improvement in functioning could make the difference between being invalided at home or getting out into the world. Often that could be achieved by morally mobilizing patient and family caregiving and tinkering with the patient's life circumstances along with his treatment regimen.

Dr. Willis Jones, as I will call him, was an elderly primary care physician from a rural town in eastern Washington State. For more than a decade, he had been plagued by excruciating pain in his upper back, the result of degenerative arthritis in his cervical spine. In pursuit of pain relief that multiple kinds of medicines had failed to achieve, he had undergone four surgical procedures, which had left him with limited ability to raise his arms and very little improvement in his pain. With the most anguished and weary expression on his face, he described the worst pain to me as fifteen on a subjective pain scale of one to ten!

Dr. Jones's wife, also in her late seventies, and their two adult daughters had come with him to the pain clinic. I remember entering the interview room where the family was waiting. Dr. Jones was seated in a straight-backed chair, wearing a neck brace and a collar pillow, his arms resting on foam rubber supports. He was dressed in a loose-fitting checkered shirt. The expression on his sharply angular face was sober and alert, his eyes fearful. His wife and his daughters also sat up straight-backed with much the same air of fearful apprehension.

A tense silence hung in the room, as if all four of them were waiting for something awful to happen. My immediate impression was of an entire family confined in a prison of pain and terrified of anything that could make it worse. As we spoke, I learned I wasn't far wrong. Pain *was* their family, they repeated. I listened as his wife and daughters described the excruciating pain that radiated from his neck into his upper back and arms, and I had no doubt they, too, had become possessed by that pain. They all seemed to be walking on broken glass, sure that some emergency would engulf them all at any moment. They couldn't stand the tension, and neither could I. Even in the space of that initial hourlong conversation, I could feel their pain finding its way into my own body.

Dr. Jones's total absorption in his pain and fear left him utterly oblivious to what his family members were going through. For their part, the family was so frightened of making things worse for him that they didn't dare discuss their anxieties with him. Their caregiving responses had actually become part of the pain— amplifying its power rather than diminishing it. We don't usually think of caregiving this way, but generations of family therapists have shown us it happens, and not infrequently. The entanglements of our relationships become so intimately associated with our symptoms that they become almost bonded in our illness experience. I once introduced the awkward term sociosomatics to explain this process. The term commonly in use, psychosomatics, seemed inadequate to me because it left out the very social processes at work, centering squarely on the patient and ignoring the environment. Whatever we call it, amplification of symptoms is real and influential, and dampening symptoms is just as real and influential. In this case, therapy for the whole family, along with drug treatment for Dr. Jones's underlying depression, produced a modest reduction in his symptoms. That small improvement made a huge difference, though, for Dr. Jones and his family, allowing them to break out of the vicious cycle and reestablish just enough normal function in their family to experience a more adequate life.

I evaluated hundreds of chronic pain patients and treated dozens more, usually in collaboration with a team of pain specialists, psychologists, nurses, social workers, and physical therapists. I conducted research on patients with pain and also those with chronic fatigue syndrome, depression with somatization (where physical complaints predominated), stigma, end-of-life conditions, and a variety of serious disabilities.

I was learning that wherever they came from, there was a lot in common among patients experiencing chronic pain, fatigue, or other symptoms and disabilities that their doctors believed were not explained by the degree of disease or injury they could document. These patients, like Jennifer Williams, felt they were treated with disrespect and disbelieved. They were often enraged by physicians and other health professionals who couldn't or wouldn't accept that they were having a serious experience with illness, or acknowledge their genuine suffering. The response required of their professional caregiver didn't fit comfortably into the caregivers' unhelpful role of policing the borderland between illness and normality. To function as real healers, those practitioners needed to affirm and acknowledge their patients, their experiences of suffering, and their desire to be successfully treated. Only this kind of respect—a deep regard, really—could reestablish trust. They needed to act as caregivers, not gatekeepers, who were ready to mobilize patients and families emotionally and morally.

At twenty-eight, Linda Howe had been suffering with chronic fatigue syndrome for two years. A medical technician, she had been worked up for dozens of possible diagnoses, from Lyme disease to early-onset multiple sclerosis, fibromyalgia, malingering, and eventually depression, which is what brought me into the case. She was caught up in a terrible relationship with her family medicine physician, who she knew did not trust her or believe there was anything "really wrong." The doctor's suspicion and doubts had spread to her family members, whom she felt she could no longer count on for genuine sympathy and practical support. The simple fact that I believed what she was saying stunned Linda.

"Your symptoms are real," I told her. "This is something you are experiencing and the fact that your doctors can't find the biological basis is not your fault. I understand how terrible this must be for you. To feel you are not being believed is to deny the reality you are going through. The suffering is real. We just don't understand yet how to diagnose and treat it in medical terms."

I wasn't surprised when she burst into tears. Nor was I surprised that after I got her physician and family to join me in acknowledging and affirming her condition, her complaints and symptoms, and the problems that they caused, slowly subsided. Regardless of what the biomedical problem turned out to be, Linda suffered from an absence of caregiving. Care was the answer.

I saw many such patients. For most, these simple caregiving acts of acknowledgment and affirmation turned out to be too little, too late. The great problem in chronic pain management, as I have indicated, is how the caregiving relationship contributes to the patient's disability. As I've already showed, the failure of caregiving has been a contributing factor in the current epidemic of drug abuse; a practitioner's feelings of helplessness come up against the sense of responsibility to do something, anything, to alleviate symptoms, and often leads him to prescribe a powerful medication, and another, and another. The outcome is drug dependency. But this failure in medical practice is not just true for pain; it holds for virtually all chronic conditions. It's not hard to see how a doctor chooses expediency rather than investing the time and attention that real care requires, and how that damning choice can add to a patient's problems.

Other patients illustrated for me other deficiencies in caregiving. But too often, the referral to a psychiatrist meant that a medical professional was basically blaming the victim, when the real culprit was poor or inadequate caregiving. Physicians and health professionals shouldn't shoulder all the blame, though. Families, too, can fall short when it comes to caregiving, adding to the burden patients experience. And the family's caregiving can also be improved.

Vanessa Jackman was a sixty-five-year-old architect and grandmother whose husband, Robert, ten years older, had survived a stroke that damaged his speech and ability to walk. Vanessa confided to me that she simply could not accustom herself to Robert's infirmities, which slowed him down so much that she lost her patience with him whenever they ventured into the world beyond their large suburban house. Robert's speech impairment and plodding gait frustrated her, and her sharply cutting and exasperated responses would agitate him and make his difficulties even more pronounced. Her own troubled awareness of this dangerous dynamic made her feel guilty, which Robert recognized, making things even worse. Their caregiving dynamic had become a painful downward spiral and upset her to the point that she stopped going out with her husband, leaving them even more trapped and isolated.

I treated them both for depression, with both medication and talk therapy, but once again it seemed to be their honest dialogue about their local world that opened a pathway to improvement. The talk therapy focused on how their caregiving and other aspects of their relationship needed to change and what that change needed to be about. Vanessa needed respite—time out and away—and also had to master her emotional response to her husband's limitations. Robert, too, needed to work on ways that he could help reduce the frustrations in their relationship. Six months later Vanessa acknowledged that those small changes had made all the difference in their lives. Again I learned that a clinician needs to address the caregiving relationship as a critical part of the illness experience, in order to help patients and families transform both.

Anxiety, as it is now well known, can be contagious. When a truly anxious person enters a family or a clinic, everyone who comes into contact with him begins to feel anxious too. We saw this at work in the cycles of pain experienced by Dr. Willis Jones and the disability of Vanessa Jackman's husband. Anxiety can make an asthmatic adolescent go into a crisis; controlling that anxiety can help her manage that crisis. (Dr. Ben was not wrong!) Depression seems to work in a similar way: experiences of loss and failure can trigger feelings of helplessness or ineffectiveness and erode a person's self-confidence. These moments of doubt and hopelessness in turn exhaust and overwhelm our reserves, worsening the depression. This regularly happens in caregiving. During my years in Seattle, I treated many family caregivers for depression—people who were loving caregivers for family members with end-stage diseases like chronic congestive heart failure, kidney failure, and terminal cancer for whom the caregiving itself had created or worsened their depression. This vicious cycle reduced their ability to give their family member care, causing the caregiver to drop out, burn out, or at the very least make the caregiving more trying and difficult. Even in the 1970s, it was known that treating patients for depression could decrease their pain and suffering and make adhering to challenging treatments more bearable for them. But I was learning that it also improved their family caregiving, which in turn helped foster better situations for their dying family members. Clearly, professional carers like me could contribute not just to our designated patients but to the nexus of care that sustained them and helped them to endure.

The more cases I encountered over those six years, the more I was able to work out the dynamics of family caregiving and to study how to strengthen them. In addition, I had put myself in a better position to appreciate the strengths and weaknesses of professional approaches to care. I published these results on strengthening the treatment of patients with chronic illnesses by dealing with depression and anxiety and improving the quality of caregiving relationships. In doing so I helped shape both the rising field of medical anthropology, by making anthropology more relevant to the clinic, while pointing the way to new clinical approaches to care, especially primary care under the then "holistic" and now "patient centered" models. My star was on the rise, and I chased after it with everything I had. Leon Eisenberg lured me back to Harvard. He persuaded the university to offer me an opportunity as a tenured professor, dividing my time between

Harvard Medical School and the Harvard Faculty of Arts and Sciences. In the medical school, I was asked to build the Department of Social Medicine around my work in the United States and Asia. In Arts and Sciences, my mandate was to build a robust program in medical anthropology at the undergraduate, MA, and PhD levels as well as with postdoctoral fellows. This conferred on me the legitimacy, along with the resources, to build what over the decades would amount to a "Harvard School" that integrated medical anthropology, social medicine, and increasingly, global health. And I brought impressive colleagues, Byron and Mary-Jo DelVecchio Good, to Harvard to collaborate with me. I came to realize that our sustained, multifaceted, and collaborative process of building research and training programs motivated me as much as clinical work.

I was fortunate to be able to continue doing clinical work as well, and I saw increasing numbers of patients. Some of them were academics. Some were Chinese with limited English-language skills. Some were referred because of problems they experienced in caregiving—professional and family—as by now I had developed a reputation as someone deeply interested in the caring condition. Still others came my way because they had various chronic medical conditions combined with depression and anxiety or histories of trauma. From these encounters, I was gaining a broader and deeper understanding of the US health care system, and the great changes that were creating havoc for patients and caregivers, including doctors.

The people I saw complained about insurance companies that put up barriers for getting the care they signed up for; about health plans that stalled in responding to claims and inquiries; about medical facilities that showed more interest in the business of health care and their legal liabilities than in caregiving. People also complained about the ever-shrinking amount of "quality" time that clinicians spent with them, and about the poor quality of explanations of disease pathology and treatment options. Others reported that their professional caregivers exhibited the sort of inattention and haste that they associated with employees of large institutions like the postal service, the courts, and big businesses.

Among the many examples was Bill Bright, a middle-aged electrician who battled a hospital and his health insurance plan for several years about charges for gallbladder surgery that far exceeded the community average for such a procedure and left him with a large debt he had trouble paying off.

Another case involved Elisa Crosby, a middle-aged African American widow who had fallen, broken her hip, and was recovering in a rehabilitation hospital. She had to appeal to a lawyer to negotiate with her health insurance plan and with the rehabilitation center to allow her enough time in the program to be able to walk independently with a walker.

Carla Miles, in her early thirties, had suffered brain injury after falling down a flight of stairs in the rural Midwest. Her injury left her with serious cognitive impairment as well as difficulty with balance that impaired her walking. There was no long-term facility willing to take her, other than nursing homes that were more like storage facilities for elderly and dying patients, rather than places where she could receive real care. Yet she was still active, engaged in conversations and relationships, and she cried (as did her parents) as she imagined living out her life in a nursing home. No assisted-living facilities, halfway houses, or other options were available. Staying home with her parents, both of whom still worked, was also not an option.

Greg Mathew, an uninsured high school dropout who worked in construction as a general laborer, went bankrupt and became transiently homeless after Medicaid denied his claims for highly expensive cancer medications. He told me that he spent much of his time battling state bureaucrats over his denied claims.

And these stories went on and on.

Over the years, hundreds of patients and families have complained to me in the clinic, at home, in research settings, or online about the poor quality of their communication with doctors. John Sales is one, a sixty-year-old teacher who went into the hospital for a surgical procedure for colon cancer. Discharged from the hospital after four days, he returned home with several drains leaking fluids from his abdomen, but neither doctors nor nurses had explained to him or his family that there would be drains. They were surprised at this development and didn't know how to deal with them. Sales's wife, his primary family caregiver, whom I was treating for depression, expressed her great fear that she would cause a life-threatening infection or some other damage.

Sarah Carr, an elderly widow suffering maturity-onset diabetes and congestive heart failure as well as a chronic anxiety disorder, developed panic attacks from a medication that no one had warned her could have such side effects. And when it was clear the problem came from her new medicine, no one apologized, explained what had happened, or took the trouble to explain about the medicine given her to replace it.

Ida Schwartz, a fifty-five-year-old nurse with acute exacerbation of chronic lower back pain, told me that an orthopedist had recommended back surgery without explaining why or answering her questions about risks. In contrast, a chiropractor had spent an hour talking to her about her problem. She didn't doubt the orthopedic surgeon was more scientific, but she believed the chiropractor was more of a healer. I could add my own story to this list. After a thyroid scan that, thankfully, ruled out cancer, neither the technician who did the procedure nor the radiologist who interpreted it were able to explain the value and limits of such an imaging procedure.

These are problems that doctors themselves lament. All in all, they reveal a sad picture of the quality of therapeutic relationships and communication in today's medicine. Yet the quality of those interactions—how clinicians listen, explain, respond to questions, relate to patients, and handle the ongoing interactions—is in fact the closest measurement we have of the real quality of the care patients receive.

Medicine in the 1940s and '50s was something like a small-scale artisanal activity practiced by individuals in solo practice or in small groups. Think back to Dr. Ben, my childhood physician, who came to our home, engaged with the entire family as individuals and as a unit, and became part of the fabric of our community. Medical practice took place in the office, the hospital, and the home, without any overarching system that governed it. In the 1960s and '70s, big business and big government began to take over whole domains of practice, conglomerating and forcing primary care, specialties, diverse technological services, and just about every kind of treatment intervention into one many-tentacled system. These powerful institutions converted physicians and nurses and the other health services personnel from independent professionals into a vast army of wage-laborers. Health care became a product. Hospitals and clinics produced it, and patients consumed it. Big medicine helped generate a big medical-legal system to respond to increasing patient complaints about their experiences of bureaucratized health care. Litigation flourished to such an extent that practitioners ran scared, spent millions of dollars on insurance, and found refuge in algorithmic best-practice guidelines (simplistic one-size-fits-all cookbook recipes).

By the 1990s and 2000s, researching evidence-based interventions on the computer replaced experience-based clinical caregiving with the actual patients. Statistics counted more than wisdom. Practitioners spent more time on the phone, speaking with insurance company representatives and health plan bureaucrats, than they did talking with patients. Corporate medicine employed the same tools corporations used to respond to unhappy customers and to attract new customers. Trainers, based on experience with airline flight attendants and restaurant waitstaff, taught health professionals how to simulate emotions like empathy. They talked about "resilience" as if patients and family carers were rubber bands who would spring back into their original shape no matter how cruel and severe the physical and emotional assault they endured. Viewed as customers, patients were socialized to evaluate health care purely in economic terms of efficiency and cost. Physicians, in response, picked up the same language and ditched the language of medicine as a moral calling and care as a moral responsibility. And so on and so on, until we have arrived at the dire straits we are in today, where there is cause for a real fear that caregiving—on the deeply human level where it matters most—could disappear from professional practice and become more highly constrained even within the formerly protected space of families and friendship networks. Patients and caregivers alike felt besieged, as if they were losing their safety net, their "haven in a heartless world," as the late Christopher Lasch, a historian of twentieth-century America, put it. Something was happening, and happening fast, to the US health care system, creating a rapidly fragmenting and increasingly chaotic and dysfunctional non-system.

Joan and I were largely oblivious to these large-scale forces and their real-world effects. These were the prime years of our life. Our children were growing into their own. Joan had found her own great mentor in the person of Achilles Fang, the sinologist at Harvard's Yenching Institute who dominated literary and literary history studies of China then. It was Mr. Fang who set Joan the task of translating *The Thousand Character Classic,* the poem in which no Chinese character was repeated, which told the story of the origin and significance of Chinese values so concisely it was used to train children in that moral tradition.

Her intellectual work was taking off, even as she looked after me and the family and as my career was exploding in every possible direction. I chaired and held named professorships in the Department of Social Medicine and the Department of Anthropology. I cranked out books and articles at an alarming pace while serving on boards, committees, panels, and organizations all over the world, and I still managed to spend time each year working in China. For almost two decades, when I was in Cambridge, I also conducted clinical teaching rounds in one of the Harvard-affiliated hospitals while seeing private patients at night and on weekends in my university office and in my home office as well. Simply put, the workload I took on was overwhelming, greater even than what I had shouldered in Seattle, and it included new administrative and teaching responsibilities. The pace was relentless, yet I didn't want it any other way. As this exciting and rewarding career achieved its high trajectory, the question again arose of whether or not I could sustain it. Clouds gathered; I wasn't prepared to accept that success and satisfaction did not necessarily go hand in hand. Every new accomplishment seemed only to drive me harder to achieve more, but that "more" didn't make me feel more satisfied.

All this would eventually have a price. Inevitably, and ironically, I would pay for my unrelenting pursuit of academic achievements and recognition with my most important resource: my health. I developed a whole constellation of ailments, most of them stress-related—asthma, hypertension, gout, sinusitis, dysplastic moles, chronic dermatitis—all exacerbated by my absolute obliviousness to the need to care for myself.

Yet it was actually Joan, not me, who shouldered a superhuman burden in those years. I wasn't quite as spoiled as in my childhood—because I did wash dishes and set the table—but my privilege was still incredible, in hindsight. I never made the bed, paid a bill, or tended to the house. I knew where our washing machine was, but I certainly had no idea how to use it, or the dryer. I pursued each and every academic and professional avenue with equal vigor and commitment but could do so only because Joan kept everything around me humming smoothly. In all this time, and after all the writing and teaching I had done on the subject, I had no clue about taking part in the care of my family and even myself. I didn't even stop to consider the social factors in my own local world that contributed to an experience with illness that I only wanted to ignore. I was harsh and demanding of my students and colleagues, constantly insisting that they do better, but hardly ever having the time and patience to delve into whatever issue might have been affecting their performance. Joan, who early on had committed to my professional success as much as I had, was my buffer, my mediator. Just as in Seattle, at Harvard she stepped in and smoothed over many of the problems my carelessness might have created.

We simply didn't have the money to hire cleaners or any other helpers. We barely scraped together the funds to pay the tuitions for our children's private schools. In the household, Joan did everything. Before we sold our house in Seattle, to make it more attractive to buyers, she rented the equipment to steam old wall-paper off the walls surrounding the house's steep stairwell. The job exposed her to toxic fumes that made her cough and feel dizzy, but she persisted and finished it. Yet just before this she had spent six intense months writing an original summary of our work in Chinese for a leading Chinese psychiatric journal. Incredibly, she was still *there* for me, for Peter and for Anne, not to mention for my mother, and even for our huge and demanding dog, Salty.

Joan played the role of primary carer in my life, and in the life of our family. She was the proverbial glue that made it stick together, while I was unwittingly doing so much to shake it all apart by charging off in my own direction. Today I must face the pathetic irony of my having written a book like *The Illness Narratives*, and having lectured about caring for people and memories, while I left it to Joan to create the narrative of our lives, and to turn our experiences into sustaining memories. These were the roles into which we had long settled. Then Joan got sick and our little world was turned upside down. This happened just as the wider world of suffering and care itself was undergoing a deep social transformation. Joan and I would come to experience some of the very problems I was documenting and criticizing. The water we were in was heating up but hadn't yet reached a boil.

Seven

It began insidiously. In her late fifties, Joan started to complain of problems with her eyesight. She had trouble reading the computer screen, or books and research articles, and frequent changes in her eyeglasses prescription didn't seem to make things better. We had developed a routine on our weekend trips from our home in Cambridge to our retreat on the central coast of Maine: Joan would read the *New York Times* to me while I drove. Inexplicably, she found she couldn't quite get through the articles, which frustrated us both. We worked out over a few months that her eyes seemed to jump ahead at the end of the printed lines, confusing the transitions between lines so that the story line itself became tangled and incomprehensible.

The frustration she felt on weekends soon carried over to the workday. She seemed to lose her command of the computer, skipping key steps, sometimes repeating the same mistake over and over again. Driving home from work, which she had done regularly for decades, Joan found she couldn't stay within the driving lanes. One unforgettable day, as we drove under the short tunnel connecting Cambridge Street to Harvard Square, which Joan had navigated hundreds, even thousands, of times, she panicked and said she couldn't drive forward in the darkness. With cars honking behind us, I was forced to reach for the steering wheel and guide the car from the front passenger seat. The episode left both of us feeling shaken and confused. From that day, she refused to drive again. It wasn't much longer before even walking downstairs and crossing the street seemed to intimidate her.

There had been other problems. She dropped a few wineglasses and dinner plates—this was unusual. A host of routine chores she had done her entire adult life now flummoxed her. First, she complained that she could no longer read bills clearly. Then she gave up writing checks altogether, turning this responsibility over to me after thirty years. I grumbled at first, but once she showed me the problems she had working out the figures, I began to sense that maybe this was more than a visual problem. I didn't push the point, because I found that I actually enjoyed taking over a responsibility I should have shared long before. We had always drunk a glass or two of wine with dinner. Joan began to complain that the wine made her dizzy. On one occasion, after a dinner party where we had drunk a fair amount, she fell asleep immediately after our guests departed and slept right through the night to late morning, something that had never happened before. And then there was the matter of our address book. Joan couldn't find listings of names of good friends and family members. She started new books for additional addresses and phone numbers. The books proliferated, but when I looked up names and addresses I found they were listed again and again in each of the small notebooks she used for this purpose. What were we to make of that?

For months, we played down the significance of these difficulties. We attributed these changes to the normal process of aging.

The only problem with this explanation was that Joan was not yet sixty. Even my ninety-year-old mother wasn't having this degree of difficulty with the familiar tasks of her life.

Then one weekend, a true disaster forced us to come to terms with what was happening. It was Saturday morning. We set out for our regular weekend run around Fresh Pond, a block from our home. Joan ran ahead, while I stopped to retie my running shoes. Loping across the middle of the wide, two-lane street, Joan failed to register the pickup truck coming from her right. I yelled, just as she screamed from the pain of the wheel running over her foot and knocking her to the ground. We both realized how close she had come to being killed and held each other as she shook from the trauma. It required two titanium screws to stabilize her fractured ankle. I stayed with her in the hospital for most of her first night there, because nothing could relieve her fear that something terrible was happening to her: the loss of her vision, her judgment, her basic competence, her fundamental sense of safety.

Our primary care physician, whom we both trusted completely, and who had been our doctor over the past several decades, was also perplexed and finally decided to refer us to specialists. First, we saw an ophthalmologist, who ran a bunch of inconclusive tests. I have a vivid memory of him casually turning his back to us in the examination room as he filled in information on the computer screen. He didn't seem to see us as real people with real lives—an unsettling sensation we were to have often, in many different doctors' offices, over the coming weeks and months. We moved on to a second ophthalmologist, who detected problems in Joan's visual fields that led him to refer us to a neurologist. This older clinician confused us with possibilities, none of which seemed to be borne out, or even connected, to his physical exam or the laboratory tests. This neurologist mumbled his way through a lengthy list of potential diagnoses, which he could neither confirm nor deny. Even with a medical degree, I was at a loss to make sense of what he said. Rather than clarifying anything for Joan and me, he only raised more questions.

Concerned friends got involved as well. One arranged for a visit to a neuro-ophthalmological unit. We waited for hours before seeing not one, not two, but half a dozen specialists. Several got frustrated at their seeming inability to slot us into predetermined diagnostic categories. Others told us that Joan was a "fascinoma," an unusual and fascinating case most likely resulting from some rare condition. This particularly angered me, as it so clearly revealed their focus on the specifics of the disease, as if that somehow existed separately from us, the patient and her husband. Meanwhile, they continued to order new and different tests and to repeat tests that had already told us nothing. Each new expert or facility, certain that they could only trust their own test results, made Joan endure the same CT scans, MRIs, and blood tests that all the others had already ordered.

By then we had spent months telephoning and waiting for appointments, having appointments changed and canceled, visiting laboratories for blood tests, going back and forth to radiology suites for new and ever more costly scans, consulting with experts who called for more expert consultations, and just plain waiting. So much of health care is about waiting, always waiting. Patients and families sit endlessly in waiting rooms, which of course only ratchets up their anxiety and frustration. They wait for results of tests, and wait to speak to doctors about next steps. Mostly they wait for answers. For people caught in the grip of this cruel cycle, waiting represents lost time, time needed for all the other things that enable us to cope, to carry on, and to prepare. The waiting, along with the frustration, multiplies, almost becoming self-perpetuating. We felt trapped in bewilderment and impotence, seen by processions of specialists who seemed oblivious to our fears or indeed our personhood. This is a piece of the illness experience that I hadn't fully understood before we began to live it ourselves.

Well-intentioned friends inevitably added to our confusion by sending us articles, referring us to websites, and sharing their own frustrating and demoralizing experiences with the health care system. Much of the information that came our way or that we looked up ourselves turned out to be contradictory and unhelpful or worse. As word spread among my former students, one, then a researcher at an institution in Eastern Europe, recommended a local healer in the former Yugoslavia who could "see" diagnoses and also could succeed in treating problems that physicians could not. As an anthropologist who had always resisted elevating Western biomedicine above other traditions and practices, I was tempted. As Joan's husband, however, I realized we weren't ready, if we ever would be, to explore this kind of unproven, even extreme, path. And, of course, our Chinese friends were recommending diagnostic evaluations and treatments by traditional Chinese medicine practitioners, which we were more inclined to take seriously, based on our past experience. Still, we hoped we had not yet reached that point. We desperately needed clarity. We needed answers.

The early stages of a serious illness are ground-shaking and universally traumatic, and even with all our purported knowledge and experience, Joan and I were not immune to the trauma. We felt overwhelmed by uncertainty and the chaos of our suddenly medicalized existence. In the often careless world of corporatized health care, so many medical professionals and their staff members seemed to see us as little more than a set of inconclusive test results and data points, rather than as vulnerable people in need of support and desperate for reassurance. We couldn't formulate reliable expectations. Although I was on the faculty of one of the world's most prestigious medical schools and was well known at its hospitals, we had no idea, nor did we receive any advice about, what steps to take next.

Finally we went to see one of my colleagues at Harvard Medical School, a senior clinical neurologist who was justly famous for his diagnostic skills. He repeated key neuroradiology tests, while methodically carrying out his own set of detailed neuropsychological tests. Finally, he sat us down and somberly went over the results. On the latest brain MRI, read as "normal" by the neuroradiologist, he detected, when compared with earlier studies, the faint but certain evidence of early cortical atrophy—a degeneration, almost a withering, of cells in an area of the brain related to visual and cognitive processing. The neuropsychology tests revealed subtle but replicable evidence of cognitive problems, and those problems, along with an exhaustive physical exam, pointed in one direction. We remained silent as my usually dry and witty colleague gravely marshaled the unmistakable evidence that Joan's troubling symptoms were caused by early-onset Alzheimer's disease. He noted that only in about 5 percent of cases did Alzheimer's begin in the brain's occipital lobes, responsible for interpreting and integrating what the eyes see. Joan was in that 5 percent, and there were already signs that the nearby parietal lobes, which help regulate sensation and perception, were involved too.

This greatly important diagnostic step completed, my senior colleague hesitated to say anything else. He could not be drawn out on the prognosis: what we could expect and in what kind of time frame. He had, in fact, no recommendations at all to make about how we should proceed. Instead he referred us to a junior colleague who specialized in Alzheimer's. In retrospect, what was most telling was that of the almost two hours we spent with him, 99 percent of the time was taken up with the diagnosis. Almost no time, after his diagnosis was clear, went into a discussion of what for us was now most at stake: What were we to do?

The neurologist's junior colleague spent most of our initial meeting encouraging us to enter a research trial, but she, too, had little to say about what we should expect and what practical assistance we should begin to look into for the future. She wanted to see Joan every six months, but told us this in a way that made it sound as if she would merely be an observer of what happened, not someone we could count on to guide us through the journey to come. She directed her remarks to Joan, pointedly avoiding eye contact with me. I let her know that I appreciated her going out of her way to emphasize that even though impaired, Joan was (and should be) an autonomous decision maker, but I explained that Joan wanted me, her husband, to help her make sense of what was already a complicated medical condition. Joan, who had been quiet throughout, spoke up and told the neurologist that she was confused and needed me to help her understand what to do. I pointed out that we wanted to go through this difficult time as a team, much as we functioned in the rest of our lives and had done so for decades. This young physician responded that "the rules" required that Joan be the one she address and also that she had plenty of experience with cases in which the husband suppressed the voice of the wife. Joan and I both said that this was not the situation in our marriage. The neurologist stood firm. We came away angrily shaking our heads, wondering how we would negotiate our future consultations with an expert who was unwilling to treat us as a family unit but only as isolated individuals. Clearly, she was following rules that were meant to be progressive, but she was applying them in a doctrinaire manner that undermined their value for us. As for treatment, she said only that the available drug therapies had not been proved to make more than a modest difference, but at least they would do no harm and might slow down the disease's progression while we waited for a medical breakthrough. On this point, it was hard to disagree. As for caregiving, she had nothing to say at all.

The night the diagnosis was made, I held Joan tightly in my arms and fiercely expressed my determination to do all I could for her, while she wept bitterly and grieved in anticipation of what we feared lay ahead. She angrily lamented that the golden years before us, which we had done so much to prepare for, were going to be something utterly, unspeakably different. I promised to take care of her no matter what happened, and that she would always be cared for at home. She was having none of it. There would be no sugarcoating. Finally, just before we fell asleep, she took my face in her hands and turned it toward her, looking directly into my eyes. I could see in her face that she was clear-eyed, sober, and determined. She spoke firmly, in measured tones, words that I never had to work at memorizing, because she repeated them over the years with the same grim seriousness. They are forever etched in my soul.

"I will not linger. I will not die without dignity. You and Charlie [our primary care doctor at that time] will know how to bring it to an end. You must promise me. I need your promise."

I listened. I signaled that I heard her request, but I knew even then that there would be little that I or her doctors could actually do. I cried with her. For her. For us both. But I was at a loss. No: I knew in my bones that no matter what we went through and what she asked of me, I could never take her life. We would together (I thought, but could not bring myself to say out loud) endure, even the unendurable.

Alzheimer's disease rarely if ever follows any kind of conventional story arc. There is a beginning, to be sure, and an inevitable ending, but the middle—the long struggle during which care comes to the fore—is for most patients and families an ill-defined and often incomprehensible jumble. The various experts and authorities on Alzheimer's tend to write about the disease as if it progresses neatly in clearly delineated stages, beginning with the early days of mild severity, the middle phase of moderate severity, and the final stage of the most serious disablement. I'm sure that kind of compartmentalization makes it easier to process and discuss the disease, but our lived experience of it was nothing at all like that. Our own illness narrative was in no way linear; it was illogical and unpredictable, and at times felt almost completely random. The story constantly looped back on itself, filled as it was with fits and starts; with lessons learned, then unlearned, then relearned again; with experiences of tragedy and victory that occurred over and over again, like a suite of unresolved themes and variations.

Indeed, life for us would come close to being unendurable over the course of ten years, but Joan's symptoms did not, at first, progress beyond the visual problems. Slowly, over a period of several years, as the synapses in her occipital lobes continued to unravel, she became blind. She was in denial, to some extent, and she worked hard to cover up the extent of the loss and its disabling consequences. But Joan lost her vision too late in life; there was no time to learn to compensate. Her encroaching blindness meant that she could not continue her translation of, or read, *The*

Thousand Character Classic, the historically important Chinese poem used to educate children in the Confucian tradition, which she had been working on devotedly for over a decade.

This blow to Joan's scholarly life was compounded by her inability to use the computer, read our research materials, or correspond with family and friends. As time progressed, she could no longer watch films, go to the museums and art galleries that she loved, or appreciate the Chinese paintings we had accumulated over four decades and that had become such a regular source of pleasure for her. I watched helplessly as, bit by bit, she lost the deep core of values and sensibility that constituted her personhood, as all the things that made her who she was fell away.

Along with these ongoing losses, Joan also had to confront the erosion of her independence. At first, she found she could no longer trust what little vision remained to get her safely across the street on her own, which meant she couldn't leave the house or the office unless she was accompanied. Later still, she couldn't find her way around the house on her own. During a visit to our son's home, she fell down a flight of stairs she hadn't seen and broke her pelvis. After her long recovery from that frightening fall, she would always hold on to me, even in our own home.

So I became her guide. I took her by the hand, kissing it and her cheek, first just to remind her of how deeply loved she was, and later on, as her cognitive functions deteriorated, to assure her it was really me. I led her around the house where we had lived for several decades: around chairs and tables, past couches and bookshelves, from bedroom to kitchen, from living room to dining room, and from my study, where the computer and television are, to her book-lined study, filled with Chinese texts and dictionaries, French novels, and the calligraphy and Chinese painting books that in the not-so-distant past she used to copy with such joy. There, in that study with her own paintings of pine trees and rocks taped to the wall, she would paint colored lines, swirls, and fragments that became looser and more abstract as her loss of vision was matched by loss of memory and understanding, until she could no longer see anything at all. Even when she was nearly blind, painting calmed her, as did most classical music. The most heartbreaking sight for me was to watch Joan try to cover the extent of her loss of vision by rushing up to family and friends, holding on to them and smiling broadly, saying hello, but all the while facing in the wrong direction.

In these early Alzheimer's years, as I began to think of them, the pace and style of our life together began to change, taking account of our new reality. We went out less, spending more time together at home. Some friends dropped away. Others became closer to us. This would become one of the recurring themes of care over the ten years of Joan's illness: people would move in and out of our lives. Long-trusted friends would disappear and disappoint, only to resurface during a later crisis. Casual acquaintances would unexpectedly insinuate themselves as critical helpmates. The dynamics ebbed and flowed over the years, such that it is now hard to reconstruct the shifting timelines and relationships. The undeniable constants, of course, were Peter, Anne, and my mother, Marcia, who stayed in daily contact as we tried to figure out what this merciless disorder meant for our future.

We postponed travel, canceled engagements, and somehow arrived at an initial plateau that gave us the false sense that we could cope without a major transformation in the order of things, at least in our domestic life. A time would come later when we'd discover that these early constraints we put on ourselves with the intent of decreasing stress had actually walled us off from opportunities to experience happiness in the world we used to inhabit, the world of friends, scholarship, reading, music, travel, Joan's cooking, and the simple spontaneous joys of going for a run or accepting an invitation to dinner. As with so many other aspects of our life, we'd readjust our attitude and approach along the way.

Joan and I saw ourselves as a unit: she represented us in certain settings; I did in others. In the health domain, our expectation was that I would take the lead. But, as with that junior neurologist we saw, a number of the health professionals we consulted resisted my speaking for Joan. They would politely hear me out, but then quickly turn their attention back to her. She would respond by telling them that I was a physician, I knew better than she did how to represent her ideas about her experience of the illness and its treatment, especially now that she was easily confused. Occasionally she would qualify or refine what I said, but much of the time she actually relied on my speaking for her, just as I had always counted on Joan to speak for me in family settings and with Chinese and French friends. We really did think of ourselves as two pieces of a whole, with a shared sensibility. In this way we didn't conform to the hyperindividualized framing by American doctors of the stereotypes of the classic triad: the responsible patient, the family member (or members), and the service provider. Our Chinese cultural socialization intensified our sense of the two of us as one unit equally responsible for each other; while the clinicians seemed to see my interventions as controlling Joan's voice.

As she became blind, however, Joan's behavior also changed. She became easily frightened and was nervous about doing even those few routine things she could still manage. Our children each had two young children of their own by this time. The babies came when Joan could still see; yet she was hesitant to carry them for fear something untoward would happen. As they grew into toddlers and then small children, she was less and less able to play with them, or even keep up with them. On one occasion in Manhattan, where two of the grandchildren lived, we carefully walked down into a subway station, but as we talked about which train to take and the tickets we needed, Joan got separated from our group and stood rigidly still, facing in the wrong direction. Quickly and silently, our five-year-old granddaughter walked up to her, took Joan's hand in hers, kissed it, and saying, "Come on, Nana," pulled her back into the protection of our family group. Watching this scene, I thought of the Yiddish expression: When a parent helps a child, both laugh, but when a child helps a parent, both cry.

Joan, who had always had the warmest, gentlest, and kindest of dispositions, became increasingly demanding and easily frustrated. Accumulated frustration led to angry outbursts. Always kind and attentive to the needs of others in the past, she became self-protective and absorbed in her own inner world. This is not at all uncommon for people in the throes of serious illness, but it can be particularly pronounced in someone with a neurodegenerative disorder. At family gatherings at Thanksgiving and the Christmas holidays, where she had always been the central figure, she became distant and interacted so little that her silence made it seem like she was no longer part of the family. Our children and grandchildren and my elderly mother tried to break through this defensive shell, but after an initial effort to engage, Joan would drift off and regain her silent space.

My son, who was particularly close to his mother, once blew up in anger at me for not working harder to include Joan in the give-and-take of family life. I didn't blame him, because it had become easier for me to accept her withdrawal and fill in the time with my own work—a fairly typical defense mechanism for a caregiver. We were in Maine at that point, and I was complaining about having so little time for myself anymore. He attacked me—rightfully, I later realized—for being selfish, after all Joan had done for me. We argued. My daughter stepped between us to defuse the situation. Then I broke down and wept. My son and daughter reached out to me, and we all cried bitterly. They had not realized how badly their mother's deteriorating condition was damaging all our relationships. And I had not realized that I needed to depend to a much greater degree on them if I was to be able to survive the multiple demands that lay ahead.

This episode in particular stands out as a moment of great clarity and acceptance. To this point, I had been doing all the caregiving myself. Now I began to realize that this had to change. I needed the help of my adult children if we were to get through this, and also that of my mother and of friends and even more distant people around me at home and at work. I had always been so proudly independent that asking for help was among the more difficult experiences that caregiving brought me, especially in this relatively early phase of Joan's disease.

Well after her symptoms had begun to affect her but before she became seriously disabled, Joan still worked with me in our offices at Harvard's William James Hall. This made it simpler for me to watch out for her while I was doing my own work. At first the staff were very considerate and helpful as they began to understand that something was wrong with Joan. Even our students pitched in. Joan would lose her way to the toilet and back. She would need help with the telephone and eventually with everything else. For the last year there, she was able to come to work only because Harvard generously provided health aides to stay with her for the hours we were in the office during the teaching term. Impaired as she was, Joan still resented the aides' presence. They were African nurses who did not have nursing licenses in America and were working for a health services placement firm (an indicator once again of the role of minority women in caregiving in the United States). The presence of these women threatened Joan's sense of self, and she went out of her way to pretend they weren't even there. Yet without them, not only couldn't Joan have been in the office, but neither could I. Someone had to look after her all the time. Once the academic year ended, this option was no longer available.

And so we had now arrived at a key point in the downward spiral of Joan's disability when it was clear she would have to stay at home. But how could I arrange that without relinquishing my own work? Early retirement was out of the question; we needed my salary to live on and to deal with the costs that came with the progression of Alzheimer's disease.

My mother's relationship with Joan was so strong that she became an important source of support. She would come to stay with Joan for a few hours to give me respite on the weekends. If I had to attend a meeting out of town, she would stay overnight—often sleeping in the same bed to give Joan the sense of security that someone was always there if needed. It worked so seamlessly that I never felt guilty that I was imposing on her. In her nineties but in good overall health, my mother still found it difficult to contribute in this way to what we now had to think of as a *system of care* for Joan. My mother never complained, however, but rather explained that it gave her a sense of purpose in life, and she enjoyed doing it, being with Joan. This helped postpone an inevitable day of reckoning.

Experienced caregivers would have recognized that I was transitioning out of the initial crisis mode to another phase: long-term care, although at the time, I couldn't have stepped back far enough from the situation to see things that way. In fact, I was largely oblivious to the change. Still in the early crisis mode, I responded by doing more, often more than I could really handle. The strong bond of our relationship carried me through Joan's progressive blindness and her worsening cognitive decline.

I had come to feel that I was flourishing in the early stages of caring for her. I was finally giving back to Joan what she had always done for me. I remember feeling happy cooking dinner and doing the dishes. Joan's denial of how severe her medical condition was also made it easier for me. We pretended that we could cope, that the losses were not so great that we needed to make a fundamental alteration in how we lived. But that's all it ever was: pretending.

And so several years slipped by. The medicines, as predicted, made no difference. But by cutting back on my busy life, which I probably never would have done otherwise, I could spend more time with Joan, looking after her increasing needs and establishing a routine of care for her. However, one of the few truisms about illness and caregiving is that the only constant is change. Just when you think you've finally achieved some stability, the illness takes an unexpected turn, or some other social or financial factor changes, and you have to start all over. In our case, we had only just settled into a manageable caregiving routine when personality and behavioral changes surfaced. There were sudden outbursts of anger; periods when she became silent and withdrawn; frustration with the limitations on what she could get done; very occasionally, panic. These episodes first colored and then transformed how Joan related to me, making it more difficult to collaborate on the care. I recognized slowly that I could no longer carry so much of the burden of care myself. Why had it taken so long to get to this point?

Things had changed substantially since the diagnosis was first made, and we could not keep moving forward on the path we had set for ourselves. We were entering the long-term care mode for a woman who was blind, cognitively impaired, and now behaviorally unpredictable. Professional care had proved limited, but now we found that the kind of family care we had devised for the early stage of dementia wasn't going to be enough either.

Our primary care physicians—first Charlie, and later Chris—knew all of this, and more. They were an ongoing source of support for us both, engaging deeply with the minutiae of daily living, with how home care was going, and with our psychological and social well-being. Their uplifting and enduring presence provided us with something approaching a sense of security as we went through this wretched experience, knowing they would be with us until the end, no matter how bad it got, no matter what was required of them. It only became fully apparent what a remarkable gift this was as we entered the darkest hours late in the course of her disease.

In memorable contrast, neither the young neurologist who followed the progression of Joan's disease every six months, nor any of the other neurological specialists we needed as her disease worsened, showed interest in these details or the necessities of family caregiving. When I informed them about what was going on at home, they looked at me as if I had forgotten that I was a medical professional like them and that I had strayed from the medically significant conversation to something more or less irrelevant.

None offered advice about the value of a home health aide. No one told us how we might modify our home to make it more appropriate for Joan's disabilities. None speculated about how a physical therapist or a visiting nurse might help us. Nor did they deem it helpful to refer us to a social worker or therapist. My status as a psychiatrist may have led them to believe that I could handle Joan's psychological, psychopharmacological, and interpersonal issues on my own. And, in fairness, they did ask me about depression, albeit in a somewhat dismissive way. But on social services and caregiving supports, they were silent. It was the diseased brain that mattered to them, not the actual, apparently lesser, problems we were having in coping. In retrospect, this is what stands out as the most troubling aspect of the professional care we received. We might have hoped at least for a team-based approach to patients and their families, where we could be referred to other health and welfare professionals in one neurological group for their advice and expertise.

It was as if the highly specialized neurologists we consulted were unaware that for Alzheimer's disease—about which so little is known of the cause and pathophysiology, and for which to this day we possess no effective treatment—it is the family and social caregiving network that make all the difference. The medical experts for this cruel disease seemed not to recognize the need to engage in hands-on professional caregiving themselves. As no doubt was true for their other patients, we needed their experience, advice, and insight to help us deal with Alzheimer's crucible of suffering and its ramifications for daily living.

After years of caregiving for Joan, I harbored the bitter feeling that once their diagnosis had been made, neurologists, unlike primary care doctors, were no help at all and contributed almost nothing to her care. I fear that many patients and family carers struggling to cope with other neurodegenerative and serious chronic conditions must come to the same damning conclusions. Medical specialists too often treat caregiving as a foreign domain or a distant, nearly forgotten relative.

A lifetime of research, teaching, and clinical practice focused on caregiving clarified these failures for me. Our neurologists saw only the disease process, not the experience of the illness. Care for them was limited to technical treatments, and once those were exhausted, as they quickly are with Alzheimer's disease, they paid scant attention to the person's suffering. They made little or no acknowledgment or affirmation of relationships, presence, the care for memories, or any other of the basic elements of caregiving. My experiences in medical school with home visits and my involvement in field research with patients' and families' local worlds had taught me that the illness and treatment experiences were centered in these domestic spaces. Failure to take these worlds into account, I knew all too well, severely limited what medical care should and could provide. And I was watching that happen in my own life with Joan. Medicine, the profession I studied and practiced and loved, was treating Joan, the person I loved, as an afterthought.

The specialists' blindness when it came to caregiving in our case was not, fortunately, universal. There were a few stunning exceptions, beginning with our primary care physicians but including several residents and students who resisted the bureaucratic tolerance for indifference and who possessed what one nurse once called "the caring look in their eyes." That nurse was careful to point out that in most cases this kind of genuine engagement with care would last less than a year, in her estimation, unless it was reinforced. The fact that the inclination to caregiving can be lost or diminished in the institutional setting attests to the power of the health care bureaucracy and the profession to grind away at the personhood of the trainee and the practitioner.

Ironically, a few of the trainees Joan encountered had been taught by me. I could see them struggling to break through what had become routine behavior for them in the hospital, so that they could demonstrate to me and to Joan that they hadn't forgotten what they had learned about caregiving. They were not alone in that struggle. For many health care workers, there exists a real desire, and commitment, to do the right thing, even in the institutional belly of the beast where they are bullied to contain costs and to see as many patients as possible in the time allotted. We don't know nearly enough about why some practitioners fail and others succeed in connecting with patients and their families. Nor do we fully understand how specialties such as neurology (in our case) fall short, while others, such as palliative care and primary care, appear to do so much better. Is it hyperspecialization, self-selection, the way clinical services are organized, or an inability to walk for the moment in another's shoes? What we do know for certain is that if a profession values human care, as nursing and physical therapy do, then the outcome for patients and families, and even for the whole medical staff, is better.

Eight

The early stage of Joan's disease had thrust me into crisis mode, but it wasn't possible to sustain that level of alarm and uncertainty while also giving her the care and attention she required. Her dementia and disability progressed remorselessly, and by the third year, I could see I'd need a plan for managing the long-term care for a serious chronic illness.

I think that from the outset, Joan found it revelatory that I could do all the things for her and for the family that I did. Not that she doubted my love or commitment, but she'd certainly never seen any evidence that I was capable of taking care of our domestic world. At first, she would thank me with an ironic shrug that suggested that if she had known I had it in me, she would have had me pitching in a long time ago. Thanking me made her feel guilty for the burdens she was now placing on me, and she would apologize, which made me feel worse, even as she coped with all her disabilities. With time, though, this dynamic, too, would fade away.

I could never have undertaken the unremitting tasks that make up dementia care if the person needing that care had not been the core of my life and my world. I felt a deep moral and emotional responsibility to repay the life-enhancing gift of care

Joan had given me for so long. But it wasn't a sense of obligation that drove me; it was my instinctive desire to see her happy and comfortable, or at least not unhappy and not uncomfortable. Joan herself made it all possible. She somehow maintained her warmth and engagement with me, on a gradually diminishing level, for much of the decade. It outlasted her responsiveness to the rest of the world around her. That fullness animated our caregiving experience, calling forth my own liveliness, and enabling us to sustain our vital connection for as long as the dementia allowed. There were moments of personal revelation, as we learned more about ourselves together than we had ever known. The reciprocal benefit of caring was the deepening of our human experience on both an intimate and a communal level.

As we progressed further into the course of Joan's illness, she continued to help with our domestic chores as much as she could. She watched over me and coached me on what to do and how to do it. As she lost cognitive function and withdrew into herself, this, too, would cease. Likewise, for as long as she was able, Joan insisted that we remain connected to our social world, and for a few years we continued to go to dinners, parties, and receptions, until invitations began to fall off as people seemed to grow less comfortable with her disabilities. I still took her to restaurants, movies, and musical performances, even as she became less responsive. Friday matinees at the Boston Symphony Orchestra thrilled her, and the many frail and disabled elderly people in the audience made her feel less self-conscious. We maintained this ritual well into the so-called middle years of her Alzheimer's. We spent time with our children and grandchildren, and went to our vacation home in Maine when we could, but even these soul-sustaining activities became less and less possible as the disease progressed.

Joan participated in our life and our program of care as much as she could for as long as she could. Most remarkably—and most significantly—she struggled to stay positive about herself and about our life together. Until she couldn't.

Over the early months and years, we settled into a daily routine. I would wake Joan up between 6:00 and 6:30 a.m. I took her to the bathroom, handed her the toilet paper, and washed her hands, then dressed her in running pants and athletic bra for our regular basement workout. Following our workout, I led her to the bath or the shower (she preferred the former and it turned out to be easier for us), helped her undress, and helped her get in and out of the tub. At first, she managed to wash her body with soap and shampoo her hair. Later, I did that for her, and also dried her off with a bath towel, then dried and combed her hair. After that, I led her back to the bedroom, where eventually, as her condition deteriorated, I had to dress her. I picked out her clothes, checking with Joan about what she preferred. At some point, she no longer told me what she wanted to wear. The cognitive decline became so serious she would stay silent or become confused by even a simple question. So I would do what I had never done before or thought I would ever have to do: choose the dresses, skirts, pants, blouses, sweaters, and jackets for her. Still later, I would have to shop for new clothes with the help of my mother and daughter. Joan had always dressed well, and I made sure she looked well dressed, even when the Alzheimer's was advanced.

After we were up and dressed, I would lead Joan from the bedroom to the kitchen, where she would sit while I prepared a healthy breakfast. At first, she would feed herself, but later I had to feed her, which I learned to do slowly so that she didn't choke on the food or the beverage. Wiping her lips with a napkin and cleaning her hands, I would stop to consider the workday ahead, what we would need for dinner that night and the nights that followed, including what shopping had to be done and when I could fit it into our cluttered schedule. We were off on another day of caregiving and care receiving.

To watch Joan decline and have to help her with these most basic things made me feel defeated at first. But amid the sadness and frustration, over bad days and better ones, feeling broken or whole, I pushed on to accomplish whatever it took to care for her. It became a habitual part of our relationship, what she expected of me and what I expected of myself. Besides the cruel, frightening times, of which there were many, there were also long stretches when together we achieved a kind of balance and harmony. These became, as the horizon of what was possible narrowed, the best of days. Nothing special happened. Joan didn't somehow get better. The decline continued. But periodically we arrived at moments, important moments, when the caregiving and the care receiving seemed to reach an equipoise. This was simply the way it was. The pain didn't disappear. The tasks to get done didn't dwindle. Yet we were happy within the severely diminished limits set by this most troubling disease. Together, we felt at such times that we could handle it.

Joan would say to me, "See, it's not so bad!" She would grin and laugh with her whole face, while opening her arms and hands in a gesture of warmth and inclusion. In these moments, she'd reveal her readiness to deny the significance of her disability or even to deny that she had Alzheimer's disease at all. At other times, I sensed she wanted such comments to support and encourage me in my caregiving chores, about which she clearly felt guilty, especially at the outset. "You can do it, Arthur! You can do it!"

Just so, she would encourage herself: "It's not so bad. I can still do a lot of things, do most things. Don't worry about me—I'm OK!" Did she believe that? I doubt it, but she felt the words were important to keep us both going. They did, in fact, keep us going, but every time she uttered them, they broke my heart.

At our most honest moments, well before this progressive neurodegenerative disease robbed her of her insight, judgment, and way with words, Joan would simply say, "Thank you, Arthur. We can do this!" Or she would stay silent but smile weakly at me. At this point, we could still go for long walks around Fresh Pond or from our home to the Harvard Business School's campus and back. When in Maine, we could walk out along the long road to Seal Cove. Joan loved these walks, and her unseeing eyes tried to focus and see what I described, and even as she increasingly succumbed to silence, her face would shine bright with happiness. We continued to enjoy our twilight glass of wine and the presence of family and friends, but Joan seemed to retreat from the conversation even though she showed her joy in her smile.

It was these transient soft states of relative stability that allowed us to go out to restaurants, shop together, and drive out to feel the autumn crispness or spring warmth, all of which clearly gave her pleasure. As our life became more and more confined to home, which was both comforting and comfortable, I could sense that Joan was going through a change. Though quiet much of the time, we kissed often, danced, snuggled, and were at the best times still lovers. Joan was affectionate, but more and more, she responded to my kisses and caresses with a faint smile. This was good enough for me, and for Peter and Anne or my mother if they happened to visit at such a moment. And yet in retrospect it was like the slow going-out of a candle. The light faded, sometimes almost imperceptibly, but inexorably, along with her language and her responsiveness.

As I try to narrate the prolonged experience of illness and caregiving that I shared with Joan, I find myself continually challenged by the certain ineffable characteristics that I've described: the scattershot randomness, the reversals and interruptions, the shifting subplots and nonlinear chronologies. A chronicle should anchor the reader in time, marking the passage of weeks, months, and years, but as immersed as I was in the all-consuming present, time became more and more abstract and relative. Everything fades in my memory into the relative degree of Joan's impairment— mild, moderate, severe, terminal—but I cannot really pinpoint how long any of those stages lasted. In that long, dark decade, I could not see a future, nor even entertain it. Our past seemed remote, and no longer tethered to the present. Time simply passed, punctuated by moments of crisis. When Joan and I danced, we moved together, not toward any destination, but just swaying back and forth in place, in the moment. We had always been moving forward, building a future, preparing for better times. Now we simply hovered in time together, and somehow that had to be enough. And it was.

This new way of experiencing time was, however, unexpectedly liberating for me. Joan had always functioned at a less hurried pace. But in the past, whatever I did—walking, eating, even just speaking—I did as if I was always up against the clock, running out of time. Joan moved at a steadier, more considered, and deliberate speed. Time had slowed down for me only when I was with a patient, listening intently. When we first received Joan's diagnosis, I immediately feared that I would become even more frenetic and exhaust myself trying desperately to get everything done. That did eventually come to pass in the final stages of Joan's illness, but for much of that dismal ten years, as I did more and more to care for Joan and for us both, I actually slowed down, matching my pace to hers.

Over time, I simply approached life in a softer, gentler way. I came to genuinely enjoy this more deliberate experience of time, and what's more, it had a healing effect on me, easing my hypertension and improving my general well-being. Joan was now in my care, and if she was prone to stop and smell the flowers, I needed to as well. I needed to see and feel what was around us as she would, so I could explain and describe things that became harder for her to sense and experience. My need and desire to be present for her in this way transformed my own sensibility, my own awareness and sensitivity to her pain and to the world.

One of the cruelties of Joan's illness was that it denied us a critical piece of our own caregiving narrative: Joan's perspective and experience. The illness experience belongs to the afflicted, of course, and over time, the caregiver moves from the status of bystander to engaged sharer, often helping the sufferer to process it all. It is in this mutual engagement that caregiving becomes an enriching, human process. As a neurodegenerative disease like Alzheimer's robs a sufferer of cognition and perspective, the human contact becomes more elusive. It was our good fortune that Joan was able to remain positive for a long time, determined to play whatever role she could in her own caregiving, but eventually the loss of cognition means the gradual loss of self. Joan was a doer her entire life. A natural athlete, a lover of the outdoors, she brightened when in motion. Whether hiking, playing, climbing, or simply walking, she felt centered and steadied by activity. Even when she became ill, I found that getting up and moving brought some measure of peace to her, and to me. The energetic activity of Joan's mind matched that physicality, but both sides of her persona faded away, leaving me little ground for assessing her mood. She retreated inside herself, increasingly unable to share or express whatever was roiling her inner world at any moment.

This illusory period of calm and balanced care crumbled away, to be replaced by escalating anxiety and naked panic that neither I nor she could control. Her personality became agitated and unpredictable. Joan could not interpret the changes in her feelings for me, but I was aware—perhaps she was as well—that the calm was an illusion that could metamorphose at any time into panic and inner pain. She had no words for me about what was happening in her interior self, although sometimes she would complain of feeling dizzy or in other ways uncomfortable. She was less and less specific about how she felt as her dementia worsened.

Then the point of balance shifted, her problems intensified, my sense of effectiveness deserted me, and we struck really bad times. I imagined these horrible days and weeks as the result of the further unraveling of the neural networks in Joan's brain, driving her descent to another, darker stage of suffering. Her problems—behavioral, emotional, cognitive—raised the already high bar for me as her primary caregiver and undermined my confidence in my own capacity to withstand our troubles and continue to care for her. At such times, our relationship seemed to seesaw wildly as if the very ground of our love was giving way. Yet then our situation would stabilize, at least for a short while, at a different if lower level of functioning.

Just as I had taken over the checkbook and household chores, I took over everything that required reading. I read newspapers, magazines, and books to her, and these gave her joy, until her short-term memory became so impaired that she could no longer follow and make sense of what I was reading. When that happened, she became agitated when I read, so instead we sat before the TV or radio, and I interpreted stories for her. Eventually these activities, too, overwhelmed her, and this made me so uncomfortable that I stopped watching the TV or listening to anything other than music that I thought might soothe her. At that point, Joan seemed content, sitting silently while I read quietly by myself. Even this bare level of intellectual life would finally give way, because Joan became agitated by my silence. We ended up sitting together on the couch while I held her hands and spoke slowly and softly, retelling the oldest of our family's stories, hoping that her agitation would subside so that she would be ready for sleep.

When her cognitive decline became so pronounced that she could no longer get around on her own, Joan had to stay at home. While my mother helped me here, she was in her nineties and I could not expect her to stay with Joan all the time I was at work. I needed to continue working both for financial reasons and to keep me going as a caregiver. The time had come when I had to find someone to help her around the house and protect her from getting lost in her own surroundings and injuring herself. Unlike other caretakers of Alzheimer's patients, I didn't need to worry about Joan wandering outside and getting lost, because her visual impairment restricted her movement. I talked to my brother, a psychiatrist in Boston, who told me about a social worker who helped family carers locate home health aides. Through her assistance, I found Sheilah, a lively Irish American woman in her thirties who had followed her mother and grandmother into this semiprofessional caregiving field. She had experience taking care of elderly dementia patients.

This occurred at a stage of the Alzheimer's progression when

Joan could still recognize what I was trying to do, and she put up a strenuous fight about our employing Sheilah. I tried to reason with her that we had no choice: I kept explaining that I had to go to work to support us, and she could no longer stay at home alone. But she wouldn't hear of it, and she categorically refused to have Sheilah, or any stranger, stay in her house.

I knew denial is ubiquitous among Alzheimer's patients. In part, it is psychological—a defensive reaction to their loss of competencies. But it also seems to be a physiological response of the brain itself to the catastrophic unraveling of its neuro-networks, which leaves the afflicted person desperately struggling to cope with diminished memory, her inability to focus and pay attention, a broken interpretive system, and in Joan's case, blindness. These horrific losses made it impossible for Joan to be effective in ordinary life tasks, and they undermined her autonomy, ruined her judgment, and forced her to depend on others to such a degree that she felt her identity threatened at the very core. And it was. For Joan, an effective, independent woman, an intellectual who had always functioned at an elevated cognitive level, and a painter and calligrapher who relied on her cultivated eye and sophisticated sensibility, the blow was devastating.

Even after Sheilah came to work in our house, over Joan's strident objections, Joan continued to fiercely resist. She refused to acknowledge Sheilah's presence or even talk to her. Joan Kleinman, who had never said harsh and cruel things to anyone, called Sheilah names belittling her and repeatedly exclaimed in the most definitive terms that she would never accept her in her home. But we had no choice, so I continued pressing Sheilah's case, while Sheilah displayed admirable patience and forbearance, telling me she had experienced rejection before and overcome it with kind persistence. It took several difficult months, and then they made emotional contact. In another few months, they were inseparable. Sheilah worked weekdays from 9:00 a.m. to 5:00 p.m., and I was home with Joan from 5:00 p.m. to 9:00 a.m. during the week and twenty-four hours a day on weekends. On Monday mornings as we ate our breakfast of oatmeal or an omelet, Joan would repeatedly ask, "Where's Sheilah?" until she arrived. And just before 5:00 p.m. after a full day with Sheilah, Joan would do the same, repeating every few minutes, "Where's Arthur?"

It would be hard to overemphasize how important Sheilah became to us. Without Sheilah, or someone like her, I would have been unable to continue my teaching and writing, nor could I have kept up caring for Joan. The strain of caregiving would have been unrelieved, and I would likely have become depressed and dysfunctional, or given up entirely. Either would have been a disaster. Sheilah not only relieved me during the workday; the close relationship she developed with Joan greatly helped Joan get out and around. Sheilah and Joan lived life together. They shopped, went for drives and walks, saw movies and went out for meals, visited parks, met friends, went to museums, and much more. Joan not only let herself be cared for and accompanied, but greatly enjoyed her outings and time with Sheilah. The change and variety that Sheilah was able to bring to Joan's daily life eased Joan's guilt that she was a burden on me, a sense of failure and remorse that drove her to tears at times. Sheilah strengthened the relationship between me and Joan, reducing the pressure on both the primary caregiver and the care recipient, while creating a parallel caring relationship, which together with those involving my mother and son and daughter made it feasible for us to care for Joan at home. Sheilah and my family couldn't transform Joan's condition any more than I could. The disease continued its implacable course.

Caregiving for Alzheimer's dementia is never about transformative change for the better; the road runs downhill. But care can manage dementia and keep all the players (including the primary caregiver) going over the long run. And even small changes like those I am describing can sustain the relationship between the caregiver and the recipient of care, helping to prevent burnout, limit failure for both parties, and make home care feasible.

The strong relationship Sheilah developed with Joan seemed to help slow down the progress of the disease, or at least gave us this feeling, and made possible some of those moments of calm and acceptance that I mentioned earlier. These crucial victories, no matter how small they seemed in the overall picture of defeat, steadied me and kept me going. Most importantly, they facilitated a change in our perspective. Some of the limitations all of us in the family had placed on our lives now seemed misguided or at best, premature. We drew courage from small successes with Joan, and sought ways to break out of our self-imposed shell. I remember planning outings or events, from attending a party to just going out to the corner store, and wondering if Joan could manage it, or if I could, and then stopping myself with the realization that, the hell with it, we have nothing to lose. If it turned into a disaster, so be it. I'd had enough experience to cope. But maybe, just maybe, the experience could be rich with humanity, and Joan's face would light up, even for a flicker of time, with pleasure.

During the period of relative stability, in the early stage that followed Joan's acceptance of Sheilah in our lives, I began to keep a journal as a way of processing my own thoughts and emotions, and to allow myself some moments of solitary contemplation and relaxation. In it one evening I wrote a description of the positive experience of caregiving that Joan and I were able to share.

I arrive home from my office: tired, pondering the day's events and anxious about what I will find. It is 5:00 p.m. on a splendid late spring weekday in Cambridge, 2006. There is a fresh breeze and the sun is not too warm. As I enter the house Sheilah passes me on her way out. She smiles and whispers, "Not too bad. Joan didn't ask: Where is Arthur? More than 20 times."

Joan greets me joyfully with her face lighting up and her arms extended. Misjudging where I am, her unseeing eyes look behind me. I kiss her on the cheek and take her hand, the left one where her wedding ring used to rest before she began to pull it off and misplace it. [I've put it in the vault in our neighborhood bank.] I kiss her hand and lead her to the sun room where I can describe to her the state of the garden, our hidden garden, surrounded with wooden fencing and a stand of spruce trees, and containing tall pines and ancient crabapples and many kinds of flowers. She was a constant gardener: a planter, a weeder, a cultivator of plants and of people. She made our family flower . . .

Often agitated. But right now, she seems happy. And seeing her so makes me happy too. I have tasks to do— make dinner; help her eat; take her to the study so we can watch the news on the TV and I can try to explain the day's news stories; perhaps go with her for a late walk around the block; help her clean up, use the toilet, change into a nightgown, get ready for bed; respond to her questions and tell her what happened to me today; perhaps she will remember how her day went, but likely not; and help her brush her teeth and climb under the covers. I get into bed with her and hug her close. If it goes well, as it has on recent nights, Joan will fall asleep before me and I will slip out of bed, lock up, pay the bills, wash the dishes, check my emails, perhaps read today's newspaper or prepare for next day's class. And this is what happened today.

I return to the bedroom to look at her in a kind of silent contemplation. We have been married so long, and I have been caring for her now for so many years, reading her face is like a Lectio Divina [ancient practice of a slow, contemplative, prayerful reading of Scriptures]. I slowly pass my eyes over her high cheekbones and arched brow, the sculpted nose and long elegant neck as if I am reading holy script and recognizing the presence of divinity in her gentle breathing. She is still beautiful, and radiates a presence, yet with white streaks in her hair and puffy, blotched skin, looks so much older. I am so much older too, I remember. There is something special here that consoles my spirit, as if I can feel fate working things out for us. But how?

It is Joan's deteriorating condition that controls her and me too. But I don't let myself think too far ahead. I try to stay in the here and now. Many bad days have prepared me to be alert and careful; ready for the next downward spiral to descend. At least by focusing on one act at a time, I can feel as if I am exercising some control over our lives, even though I know this is merely a useful fiction.

I run through what I need to do in the next twelve hours or so. When should I wake her up during the night to go to the toilet, so that she doesn't soil herself? When do we need to get up in the morning so that she has enough time to participate as fully as she can in a workout, and then for me to bathe and dress her? Which of her medications do I need *to put out for the morning? Which clothes? Which type of breakfast? And then I look ahead to the new day's challenges. Will she awake agitated or paranoid?*

I am her primary caregiver, but I also need to keep my adult children, grandchildren, ninety-four-year-old mother, and the rest of our family and close friends up-to-date about her condition—and also my condition as her caregiver. Everyone is worried about us both. I've gotten used to the routines, but periodically things worsen and I wonder once again if I can do this. I realize that at some point, I'm not going to be able to continue. And then what? I quickly change the line of my thoughts so that I can forget that fear for the moment; forget the losses and hurt too, forget what love and fidelity require. Fortunately, there are many other things to think about. And, tired though I am, I can savor the transient calm, the tenderness, even as I steel myself to face yet another day in what has become such a long and troubled journey. So ends just one day, a good day this time, in my life as a caregiver.

Financial resources made all the difference for us. I could afford a home health aide. People with limited resources in Japan and Scandinavia also have access to this crucial component of home health care. But poor and near-poor people in the United States do not have this advantage, making care in place much more difficult, even impossible, for many.*

---

* My own state, Massachusetts, is one of the few where poor families have an alternative. According to the website of Elder Services of the Merrimack Valley, "The Community Choice program offers MassHealth standard enrollees who are nursing home eligible the choice of receiving their care at home, which can delay or prevent imminent placement in a long-term care facility. The Community Choice Program provides assistance with daily living and personal care needs. MassHealth recipients must be 60 years of age or

As Joan's neurodegeneration gradually worsened, a cycle of decline and response played itself out. This is the very hallmark of *chronicity*, the term used in medicine to describe a long-term medical condition. At each new level of Joan's impairment, it took time before I could adequately adapt and begin to feel comfortable again as a new stage of loss and struggle set in. The experience was the same for Sheilah, and for Anne, Peter, my mother, and the rest of our family and friends. We barely got used to a new limit on Joan's functioning—cognitive, visual, emotional, behavioral—when a further downward spiral would send us scrambling to find new ways to cope. The cycle was not regular. Joan's condition would worsen with different consequences for her and us, sometimes gradually, other times gaining destructive speed, and then once again slowing down and plateauing for a period. Just as I began to feel I was getting a handle on what I needed to do, things would seem to fall apart once again as Joan and I descended to what in the final years felt like the next circle of hell. Her emotions became even more unstable and unpredictable; she would alternately become sad, agitated, and easily frightened; every once in a while she displayed flickers of suspicion bordering on paranoia. As this state, which lasted for several years, also worsened, Joan developed periodic hallucinations and delusions. She would, for example, start talking aloud as if she were addressing an old friend or a family member who was not in fact present. She would also occasionally but very briefly act as if the house and its occupants were not real, as if her food was poisoned, or as if one of us was spying on her and recording her secrets.

This wild and uncontrollable state complicated caregiving

---

older." From "Alternatives to Nursing Home Care," https://www.esmv.org/programs-services/alternatives-to-nursing-home-care/. Accessed September 4, 2018.

greatly and made it more difficult to take Joan out to shop or to eat at a restaurant. She might impulsively try to open the car door while the car was moving or raise a ruckus in a coffee shop or restaurant. While in a shop, she might become agitated and demand to leave, or argue with the cashier over something nonsensical or trivial like the color of the receipt. When Sheilah and I took Joan to the local shops and places to eat where we were all well known, the shop owners, waiters, salespeople, and bank tellers would make light of these disruptive behaviors. They would normalize the episode with a laugh, a warm gesture, or a distracting story. In a real sense, they, too, became part of our caregiving nexus.

Not all of our neighbors or other community contacts at this stage showed this kind of compassion—a few walked away, muttered something hurtful, or treated Joan as socially dead, a nonperson—but many helped us in the most practical, decent, and human of ways. They gave Joan face, as the Chinese would say: they enabled her to maintain a sense that she was still part of things, and they helped protect her sense of self and preserve, even at bad times, her dignity.

It is a sad but instructive irony that this solicitous attention occurred much more frequently in our local community—at the bank, at the checkout counter of the neighborhood grocery, even at the large supermarket—than it did at the teaching hospital where she was examined every six months, and where Alzheimer's patients were coming and going on a regular basis. There the receptionists, nurses, and young physicians-in-training were just as likely to be mechanical, insensitive, and lacking in simple courtesy as they were at other times affable and supportive.

And yet I saw the same failing at times in myself as I struggled with the burden of adapting and caring. It was hard to maintain an encouraging attitude for long, long stretches of time when Joan was so cognitively and emotionally impaired, and at times so demanding and frustrating. I cannot imagine how challenging it is for professionals to see not one but a procession of patients with Alzheimer's make that long, grinding downhill journey, to project the courtesy, decency, and helpful human warmth that dementia patients and their caregivers need so much. Without that kindness and enabling warmth, the burden of suffering becomes unbearable. Yet there is evidence to support the commonsense conclusion that endeavoring to maintain one's human presence also benefits the caregiver, whether family member or professional. It creates a greater sense of purpose, reduces burnout, and can even make otherwise emotionally draining work meaningful, at times even joyful. This was also my experience. Respite and resources helped greatly, but ultimately it came down to commitment to a particular human being, who in turn, even when impaired, contributes to keeping the relationship vital.

Conversely, when the corrosive effects of bitterness, resentment, or exhaustion come into play, care relationships can quickly become dysfunctional, or worse, sometimes cascading into cycles of verbal and psychological abuse, and even physical violence. As difficult as it may be, for their own sake and for that of their "charge" (be she kin or client), caregivers need to remain vigilant, alert to mood swings and other warning signs, not just in the person for whom they are providing care, but in themselves as well. Fortunately, I was spared such a threatening downturn, but I did on occasion become angry at Joan, usually out of my own frustration and exhaustion. When I recognized what I was doing, and reaffirmed for myself that her suffering was more important than my own, I could stop myself before I lost my temper or said something hurtful. No doubt, my psychiatric training helped me, as did the many years of Joan's influence, which softened me and opened me up to self-criticism. Most caregivers have not been so well prepared, and yet they carry on.

The literature on caregiving generally fails to consider the central role of the care recipient. The caregiving relationship involves the committed efforts of both. Joan was an active participant in her own care until the final year of her life. Her engagement enabled—and at times, disabled—the work of caring, but she was always present. At the beginning, she and I both emphasized her capacity to care for herself, since so much of her identity was rooted in her competence and self-sufficiency. As she became increasingly disabled, this diminished, although she fought hard to hold on to it. Emotional and moral reciprocity underwrote nearly every caregiving interaction. Without it there would have been little or no trust. Joan's responses to me were so warm and appreciative, so connected psychologically and physically, that they were inseparable from my own actions. When she became resistant or distrustful, as she did toward the end, caregiving became nearly impossible.

The decade during which I became Joan's primary carer remade my life. I experienced pain and disappointment, failure and exhaustion, difficulty upon difficulty. I also became a different person, a better person. I learned more about life, and how to live a good life, than at any other time. I did not become embittered or depressed, although at the worst hours I may have drifted toward despair. I never lost hope, although my hope for us and our family shifted from a focus on the two of us to an emphasis on our children and grandchildren. I can't deny that in the darkest hours, I felt devastated and hopeless, but those moments were fleeting. Caregiving made me feel both stronger and better about myself in my relationships with others. It furthered my liberation from driving ambition and from the single-minded absorption in my work. It made me learn to take care in how I lived, in how I related to my family, and in the minutiae of everyday life, which, when all is said and done, is what living is about. I took on greater cares—much greater, to be sure—yet they reoriented me to what really mattered. Some people, most often women, learn this in caring for babies and small children. I learned it from taking care of Joan. Caregiving teaches one humility: you learn that no matter how able and successful you may be in some realms—and no matter how hard you try to make things go well—stuff, bad stuff, is going to happen, and often you have no control at all over it. I learned to accept that the world could not be bent to my will and that I had to adapt, sometimes in significant or uncomfortable ways. But I learned even more than this; in my innermost being all I could really control was how I reacted, how I responded. It was this that made those years such a redeeming experience. My mother described it to Anne and Peter very succinctly: "It has made him human!"

The Chinese phrase *guo ri zi* refers to living a life of responsibility for good fortune in one's family. It is part of what it means to mature and cultivate oneself as a human being. I had failed to master this in my early life. I began to learn it from the way Joan lived life and how she cared for me and for our family. The practical lesson continued as I cared for her. I had learned to take care by giving care. Perhaps the simple truth about the transformation during this period is that I became a reflection of Joan, taking on many of the defining characteristics of the person she was before the Alzheimer's disease took hold. I had absorbed the best parts of her persona—the caring, the calming, the attention to details—maybe not with her natural grace, but certainly with her sense of purpose.

It was during this time, in the last few years of caregiving, that I undertook regular exercise, slept better, created moments of genuine self-reflection, and learned to do so in the midst of many conflicting demands. After the earlier period when my health problems actually worsened under the stress, I worked on them (and on stress management) so conscientiously that at the close of that terrible decade, I was more robust and much healthier. I also learned how to find joy in the moment, and to relax under pressure, especially in my work life. It was a period when I deepened my ties to family and friends by actively nurturing those relationships. None of this altered the fundamental reality of Joan's constant decline and the many troubles it brought our way. The dreaded outcomes all came to pass, as we knew they would. And yet in some inexplicable way, I emerged remade.

That process of becoming more fully human, and growing into a mature version of myself, enabled me to withstand, and possibly assisted Joan, too, in enduring what became the most arduous and troubled period of our life together. There is much talk about "resilience" in dealing with adversity, but for me that word carries far too positive and even triumphal a meaning. No one goes through truly serious illness, caregiving experiences, and loss without being broken and losing something of what matters most to them. "Endurance" for me is closer to my experience. Caregiving is about enduring.

Of course, as the physician and philosopher William James understood over a hundred years ago, we inhabit a "plural universe," meaning that societies, communities, families, and individuals have multiple, different, changing, and even contradictory experiences. The upshot is a large array of differing responses to life problems. Caregiving also needs to be understood as plural and diverse, in that there can be as many different experiences of it as there are caregivers and care recipients. My own reveals only so much. It needs to be extended by other stories of care that illustrate the varieties of caregiving. Each situation plays out in its own local world, with unique financial pressures, family and interpersonal dynamics, and social customs, all of which influence decision making, task sharing, and all the other key processes of care. Take, for example, my own experience with Sheilah. Joan and I would have benefited from understanding what a home health aide can provide much earlier in our caregiving trajectory. My decision to engage a home health aide was forced upon me almost as an emergency measure by the pressure of events created by Joan's worsening disability and the associated caregiving demands. There was too little time to prepare for it or to canvass available alternatives. As it was, we were so fortunate to find Sheilah. But I know others facing the same conditions who have not had such good luck. It is imperative that at the very onset of the diagnosis of Alzheimer's, physicians clarify the importance of taking this and other caregiving supports into account when planning for what lies ahead, or at least refer the family and patients to colleagues for whom this is a professional role. Our specialist doctors didn't really manage to talk to us about what was in store for us, or advise us on how to cope with any of it by reorganizing our lives and expectations.

So many caregivers confront agonizing choices, and no two situations can be the same, and yet we can find both wisdom and comfort in the experiences of others. Alice Tsai, an attractive fifty-year-old Chinese American businesswoman, was referred to me by her primary care physician for treatment of depression in the context of family caregiving. She felt desperate, trapped in a thirty-year marriage to a much older Chinese real estate developer who had experienced a series of strokes, which had left him with right-sided weakness that affected his walking and use of his arm as well as slurred his speech. He was dependent on her for help with dressing and bathing and other activities of daily living. Alice spoke bitterly of being forced to care for a husband who had refused her wish to have children, had treated her badly over many years, and about whom she had come to feel emotionally remote and resentful. The caregiving compounded her feelings of living a desolate life.

Treating her depression considerably lightened her emotional burden and enabled her to deal with what we both agreed was a moral problem. In response to that problem, she drew on the Chinese tradition, which embraces the idea that human life often ends in disappointment and failure. Nonetheless, the moral person must persist and endure, thereby elevating his or her own human qualities even in the face of bad outcomes. (I had talked with her about marriage counseling and divorce, but for her neither was an acceptable option.) She was relieved and grateful to have found a way to accommodate her situation and to endure. Hiring home health aides from a Chinese American organization also made her caregiving more feasible. I came to greatly admire her existential commitment to care in the absence of love—something I am almost certain I could not have managed myself.

A fellow medical academic at a midwestern university who heard about my work on caregiving consulted with me about the care he was giving his wife of forty years who was in the end stage of Parkinson's disease. His son and daughter, both in their late thirties, each married with small children, lived a great distance away and had been unhelpful and remote. He tried to get them involved in caring for their mother, but their lack of interest left him bitter and disappointed. He felt he could no longer care for his wife alone, in spite of having home health aides and visiting nurses. I asked him why he thought his adult children were unwilling or unable to offer help. He told me ruefully that he thought it had to do with the way they were raised: they wanted for nothing, which had made them complacent, irresponsible, self-centered, and unused to reciprocating. I suggested he speak frankly with them about all this, and make it clear how much he needed them now, but he didn't think that was possible. He lamented that he had never spoken to them this way, and didn't know if he could beg them to help him. A proud, hyperindependent, controlling father was confronting a situation he could no longer control. Realizing how my own children had responded to me when I confessed I needed them, I recommended that he express his sense of losing control and his very real need for help and request it of his children. When I later heard from him the bitter news that they hadn't responded as I had hoped, I was out of answers.

I tell this story because all of us live lives that are complex and distinctive. One must retain honest humility when offering advice. Caregiving is about relationships above all else, and troubled or failed relationships are rarely a promising source of successful care, even when supported in other ways.

A good friend spoke with me about her mother, who died in her late nineties, succumbing to end-of-life heart and brain failure. For the final two years of her life, her mother lived, with cascading dementia, in a nursing home. Prior to that, she had lived on her own for several precarious years in a large Cape Cod house, her home of seven decades from the time she married. During those uncertain years, my friend—one of three siblings, but the only one who lived in close proximity—was regularly caught up in those domestic activities her mother was willing to cede to her. Her mother had been independent following the death of her husband twenty years before and was reluctant to acknowledge that she could no longer manage on her own. Denial became a crucial problem. It took several years of increasingly difficult confrontations before her mother accepted that she could no longer live alone. By the time she was ready to face this reality, she was too impaired to be a candidate for assisted-living facilities. Once she entered the nursing home—incontinent, barely able to use a walker, her short-term memory impaired—she became much less moody and stubborn. The last eighteen months of her life, my friend reported, were among the warmest times she had shared with her mother. Hence she questioned the wisdom of the current eldercare mantra: "aging in place." She is now convinced that her mother's final years would have been far happier for them both had she transferred from the family home to an assisted-living facility sooner. At the same time, she understands that their experience was uniquely their own, just as every illness experience is unique, and the same decision in another family might not yield the same results. This, of course, is William James's point: aging, like family relationships, constitutes plural realities. A one-size-fits-all approach cannot produce tolerable alternatives for what so often is an intolerable reality. Caregiving policies, like caregiving practices, have to begin from an understanding of the wide variation in family and network relations that translates into the same variation in caregiving. Such policies also need to be based on the recognition that perhaps one-quarter of elderly Americans are living alone, meaning that there may be limited family care or none at all.

My friend's experience resonates with my own, not only with Joan but with my mother, Marcia, who died not long after Joan, at the age of 102. Until four years before, at the age of ninety-eight, she had for three decades lived on her own, entirely independent, in an apartment near Harvard Square, but it was then apparent that she was struggling to keep going. At first, she moved in with me. I felt she would be happier in a family setting she knew well. Besides, I looked forward to her company, having recently lost Joan. In reality, though, it turned out to be less than ideal. Confined to my house, away from friends, my mother passed her days growing lonely while she waited for me to return from work each evening. After several months of this experiment, my brother convinced me and her that a nearby assisted-living facility would be better for her. There she could have her own space but would be surrounded by other people as well as supported by a staff who provided meals, supervised exercise, offered social programs, and could give her assistance with bathing. An exceptionally outgoing person, my mother could both socialize and, in spite of being frail, keep some of her prized independence.

The first four months in assisted living were hard for her—so much so that she kept wondering aloud why she had to live to such a great age. "Wouldn't it be better for all of us if I died?" she would cry. She thought God had forgotten her. During this transition, it looked unlikely that she'd survive for long. She fell, breaking her femur, and wanted nothing done to fix the break. When a skilled orthopedic surgeon assured her that even if she had no wish to walk again, it would still be much easier for caregiving if she had a rod put in to stabilize her leg, she very reluctantly agreed. My brother and I and my adult children were surprised to be going along with a surgical procedure for a frail ninety-eight-year-old, but the outcome was a huge and happy surprise.

After a few months of recuperation, she was back walking with a walker. As she felt more settled in her new surroundings, her spirits improved and she made new friends. At age one hundred, she was doing better than we could have imagined. She remained spirited and engaged with world affairs, reading the books I brought and giving me her well-informed views on politics and social events. She was stronger and her emotions were more stable than they had been for years. She had occasional bad days, but she also experienced many good ones. Her interest in living revived, especially when she was with her family and close friends, whose lives in turn were enriched by the time they spent with her. The end came when she was 102; her care needs had grown so great by then that we had moved her to a nursing home, where she died. Here again is a story of variability in aging and eldercare. Family carers need to be open to the variety of later life experiences that, like so much of life, are usually based on the particularities of individual lives.

I have known several remarkable women who have raised children with serious disabilities while pursuing professional careers. One is married to an equally remarkable husband; the other two went through divorces early in their experience of caregiving. Both of the latter felt that their former husbands were unprepared to be lifetime caregivers for their impaired children. Looking back, both women recognized how extremely difficult it had been for them to give their disabled children the necessary care while sustaining their own professional careers as single parents. These two women never knew each other, but they used virtually the same words to characterize their experience of caregiving. It went something like this: "I knew I had to do it, so I devoted myself to it, completely. It was terribly difficult, but you know, I endured, and I am proud of what I have done. When I look at my son [both are young men now] I feel simultaneously stricken that he is in this condition, and I am still with him, but also impressed we have both made it this far and done what we have done. Don't get me wrong. There is no sense of victory. How can there be when so much must be done just to keep going? But I am stronger now, and the caregiving is what I do, good times and bad." In my mind, it boils down to simply this: "I did it because it was there to do."

This is more or less what the late respected *New Yorker* writer E. S. Goldman concluded about the ten years he spent caring for his wife, who eventually died of Alzheimer's disease. He had written a highly readable account of that experience, *The Caregiver*, under the pseudonym Aaron Alterra, and was giving a reading from it at Porter Square Books in Cambridge, which I attended in 2007.

A young woman in the audience, following his concluding remarks, asked him what sustained his caregiving even at the most difficult times in his wife's progressive deterioration. At ninety-four, standing bent, unsteady, and fragile, gripping a walker but still in possession of great clarity of mind and a strong sense of humor, Goldman responded in a robust voice, "It's what you do!"

"What do you mean?" his young questioner persisted.

"You do it," he added flatly, "because it is there to do. It was part of the deal—you know, the marriage vows, the way you lived your life together over the decades. You do it!"

You do it because it is there to do. Women and men have said this to me while explaining how much the care they provided cost them in dollars, deferred dreams, career, energy, and emotions. I, too, heard myself saying this many times in response to questions about my caregiving for Joan. What does it mean? That the family caregiver does not so much make a decision as acknowledge a basic reality: In this centrally important relationship, someone who means a great deal to me requires assistance and I am here to offer that care; what is more, I will keep giving care for as long as it is needed and as I am able. That's all there is to it. These responses, like those of the two women with disabled children and

E. S. Goldman, underline for me the recognition that care is an elemental action like rubbing a sore shoulder or washing dirty hands. You don't think about it; you do it. You do the feeding, bathing, grooming, and getting around, not to mention the effort put into emotional sustenance. And you keep doing it. You work at it. You worry over it. There is always something that needs doing, so you keep doing.

Seen this way, and as I saw it while caring for Joan, caregiving is an existential action affirming a moral commitment. It is one of those highly valued things so deeply at stake that it requires little thought but lots of action. You do it because it is there to do.

Things are rarely so clear-cut in real life, of course. There will come a time when you can feel in your core that you can't go on. You must escape. And there are those family members and friends who never even get started, who feel from the beginning they can't do it at all, and choose not to participate. Family caregiving can also be about the absence of care. Friends of mine are the grandparents of a young woman who works as a nursing assistant in a local nursing home for the elderly in coastal Maine. They were struck by her sobering observation that most of the elderly she assists have no visitors. Her charges explain with sadness and embarrassment and sometimes anger that their son or daughter and grandchildren live too far away and have so much going on in their own lives that they don't visit. Perhaps even more tragic are the families in which the children are nearby and perfectly able to provide care, but choose not to, because of the nature of their relationship. Or they remain silent and bitter, examples of the failure of family care.

Some family members are broken by caring for disabled members: financially, relationally, emotionally, morally. Some are making it through, but just barely, bouncing from crisis to crisis. Some are balancing feelings of guilt and bitterness; still others feel only resignation. Unstable and difficult relationships, unspoken histories, and half-buried grievances are often the hidden story line in these cases. Inadequate resources (financial first and foremost, but also cognitive, emotional, and social) provide poor sea anchors for weathering the storm of illness and care. There are no simple conclusions, and no universal answers. All we can do is dig deeply into each illness experience to identify and cherish what matters most to each individual and in each relationship.

Financial pressures overshadow long-term care relationships. Henry Wright, for example, was an affable, middle-aged, low-level employee in a real estate agency who was looking after his father, a ninety-three-year-old widowed former policeman who lived in the same house with Henry and Henry's wife. They were in the always challenging process of making plans for the elder Mr. Wright's transfer to a nursing home because of the assistance he required when a small stroke left him with difficulty showering, shaving, and using the toilet. Henry and his wife simply couldn't give Henry's father the help he needed themselves. They all agreed a nursing home was the only solution they could afford. They also agreed that given their modest means and what Medicare and Medicaid would pay for, they would accept a nursing home that in Henry's eyes was nothing more than adequate, or in his words, "good enough." They knew there would be much they wouldn't like about the place, but as long as it was safe and reasonably clean, it would have to suffice. Quality for them, as for many Americans with substantially constrained financial resources, would have to take a back seat to financial reality—and they realized that even with Medicare, what they could afford wouldn't be anywhere near what they wanted.

I knew several families of somewhat higher middle-class income who could no longer afford to pay for a disabled parent's assisted living, and in one case a specialized eldercare unit. They shifted their parent to Medicaid-accepting facilities with a significantly reduced level of assistance (fewer nurses and nurse's aides) and graciousness. They felt bad about the choice forced upon them and about the quality of care their parent would experience. But practical concerns overwhelmed their familial sentiment.

It is not just a cold economic calculus that families use to make decisions about what level and quality of care is acceptable. How that financial situation is negotiated can reflect the emotional realities and the actual conditions of family and friendship relations.

Jill Connolly was a middle-aged attorney at a New York law firm. Her ninety-year-old mother still lived in the small West Coast town where Jill grew up. Jill described her family to me as dysfunctional. Neither her younger sister (an unmarried professional in Los Angeles) nor Jill (in her third marriage with two adult children) was close to their mother—or ever was. Yet both felt an obligation to help support her, so together they paid for her residence in a cognitive care unit that was part of a large retirement complex. Jill's sister, who lived much closer, visited her mother once every few months, while Jill herself visited once or at most twice each year. She described these visits as difficult.

Because they were unable to have serious or meaningful conversations, and because her mother was impaired enough to confuse Jill with other family members, she told me in a stricken voice that she had no idea why she kept visiting, other than a vague sense of obligation. She and her sister decided that if their mother survived the next year, since she had exhausted her own savings, they would work on shifting her support to Medicaid, and move her to a less expensive but also lower-level public nursing facility. Jill told me with tears in her eyes that she didn't know if at that point she would continue to visit her mother. I came away from our conversation with the distinct impression that Jill was distraught mainly because she felt the absence of caring feelings for her mother. The emotions that motivate caregiving are not felt by everyone, and yet as in many societies, one still expects and relies on families to care for their own members. That expectation engenders in some a sense of guilt and anger about unfairness. Sometimes great guilt can cause serious problems at the end of life when family members, to assuage their unbidden feelings, insist on medical intervention that everyone else finds futile and, if anything, actually reduces the dying parent's quality of life.

One widely shared experience in caregiving for individuals with chronic progressive disabling or terminal conditions is the gathering sense of finality. The care may be long-term, as it was for Joan, yet the caregiver understands that at some point it will end. He knows that the end is coming, but he doesn't know when, and he doesn't know quite what it will look like. Its recognition can breed anxiety and fear regarding whether the caregiver can be present until the end. I remember worrying on several occasions that if Joan survived me, Peter and Anne, who had young children and active lives and lived some distance away, might not be able to care for her or, if she entered a nursing home, visit her regularly. Each of the women I mentioned who had children with severe disabilities feared greatly that when they died or became disabled in old age, their child would have no family caregiver. I personally found this idea too threatening to seriously entertain for long, and actively tried to repress or deny it. Such is the amount of detail a caregiver needs to address in the here and now, that big questions like this can too easily be put aside. Yet eventually this issue must be faced. The question itself covers the final stage of care and difficult themes like hospitalization, nursing home placement, and hospice. I knew it was a good idea to think hard about these issues well before they became a reality. But in truth I found myself dealing with end-of-life issues only when we actually got there, and that was hard enough.

Nine

I think of the late stage of Joan's illness—not the final stage, but the last stage in which I was her primary caregiver—mainly as dark times. At its worst, it was about enduring the unendurable. I've spoken with a number of family caregivers whose loved one suffered from dementia, especially early-onset Alzheimer's disease, and almost everyone recognizes that experience. The challenges start with the relatively mundane, perhaps the simple failure to feel appreciated, and rise to despair and near-total exhaustion, all of which is compounded by the looming sense of hopelessness and inadequacy in the face of the mounting tasks in front of us. Every illness experience has its own heartbreaking details, but they all share one inevitability: the bad times in caregiving accumulate fast as dementia deepens, ultimately reaching a level at which an untrained family caregiver is overmatched.

Joan was transiently agitated during much of the decade she lived with Alzheimer's disease. But now that agitation, at a relatively low level, was almost constant. We no longer had times of calmness and equipoise. Yet still, this background hum of heightened anxiety in her would periodically erupt into a state of wild frenzy. And rather than last for minutes, as it had in past years, this uncontrolled hyperactivity lasted for hours, sometimes even more than a day. During these times, Joan did not respond to efforts to calm her through words. Tranquilizers, too, had little effect. She could not be controlled, so that it felt as if all we could do was wait until the frenzy burned itself out and she flopped to the floor in exhaustion.

This truly terrible state seemed to me to be followed, and perhaps preceded, by negativity, the first manifestation of which was resistance. Instead of collaborating in the caregiving, which she usually did, she would reject care from others, at times refusing to get out of bed, or shower, or get dressed. She also made negative comments about people who were around her, which she had not done before. For example, during her week in McLean Hospital's Geriatric Neuropsychiatric Service, she could not abide several of the other patients, especially those who were loud and self-important.* Joan shouted at them that they were "crude" and "disgusting." The negativity extended to the nurses and aides, and even the doctors. She criticized them, refused their help, and repeated nasty things about them. It was so far out of keeping with her former self that I was shocked when I saw her acting like this. Neither Sheilah, nor I, nor our family members could get Joan's agitation and the dark emotions and hostile behavior under control.

Joan became prone to dramatic outbursts of anger. Periodically she would lose contact with reality altogether. There was no reasoning with her, no means to calm her down. In her worst moments, she would descend into delirium, striking out, shouting and then screaming, unresponsive to anything anyone might do or say. This is among the most confronting aspects of caring for

---

* McLean Hospital is a psychiatric hospital affiliated with Harvard Medical School and located on a bucolic college-like campus in Belmont, Massachusetts. It has a noted geriatric neuropsychiatry unit to which Joan was admitted for a short-term stay.

dementia patients, much like what caregivers of psychotic patients go through.

My memories from this period bounce around in my mind, persisting as a series of colliding moments of overwhelming distress. We were descending in the crowded elevator of an office tower in Boston's financial district after a tense and troubling meeting with our attorney. We'd begun the difficult discussion of legal affairs that arise in the course of dementia—the need for power of attorney and guardianship, health care proxy, and our wills—which had made Joan confused and agitated. She pulled away from me just as the elevator's doors opened, and was immediately knocked almost to the ground by a group of young women rushing out for a lunch break. They didn't slow down to see if she was all right, and they didn't apologize. Joan was so frightened, she froze in place and refused to move, making it difficult for me to help her get to a safe place. I was angry, not at Joan, but at the insensitive young workers who ignored an obviously disabled person.

On another occasion, we were dining out at an upscale Boston restaurant with my mother and my brother and sister-in-law to celebrate Joan's birthday. It felt good to get out of the house for an evening. As we took our seats, Joan suddenly jumped up, started yelling at me angrily, insisting she was not a child, there was nothing wrong with her, and I didn't need to help her into a chair. A few minutes later, she jumped up again and screamed when she discovered that we had not ordered wine for her, because of her doctor's orders not to mix her medications with alcohol. This time she didn't stop shouting, even after I caved in and ordered her a cocktail. She was causing a scene, disturbing everyone in the room. I had experienced this behavior before and knew it could escalate. Joan might become completely wild and out of control. I hesitated as to whether I should take her home immediately, sensing that the pressure of being in the restaurant might be too great for her, but I decided to stay. I really wanted her to enjoy this family event.

The dinner did not go well. What should have been a celebration felt more like a nervous prelude to disaster. Every few minutes, Joan erupted in a fit of temper. After dessert, a birthday cake with candles, we got up to leave, and Joan fought me over helping her on with her coat and escorting her out of the restaurant. At the door, she continued to berate me. She wouldn't take my hand as we walked to the car, forcing me to walk out in traffic to prevent her from being hit by passing cars. On the drive home, she threatened to jump out the car door and end it all. By the time we arrived home, she was wild and frenzied. She knocked over a small table and began hurling framed pictures and other objects to the floor. She had lost all control, and I feared she would hurt herself. I could barely contain my own anger, and, not for the first time, I wondered if I could go on doing this. Refusing to change her clothes or go to bed, she finally fell asleep on a couch. I covered her with a blanket, and sat in a chair for hours, wondering what to do. When morning came, she was tractable again, and had no memory of what had happened the night before. "Why did we sleep in the living room?" she asked me.

Another episode took place in New York City. Just getting there was a minor triumph. I didn't want to chance going by air, so I drove. I suppose I was overly ambitious in taking Joan to a performance of Verdi's *Don Carlo* at the Metropolitan Opera, but my cousin had bought us expensive tickets, knowing that Joan and I loved this particular Verdi opera and had seen it several times before the illness set in. During the four-hour drive to New York, Joan became agitated. When I stopped at a service area to fill up the car's gas tank, Joan wanted to use the bathroom. I couldn't imagine her doing it on her own, but fortunately, I found an elderly woman who was willing to accompany her. Once back in the car, Joan became restless and aggressive, but I was able to calm her and continue the trip. We stayed with our daughter, Anne, and that made it much easier all around. At the performance, Joan became quite anxious. Early in the first act, she started talking to me in a regular conversational voice, disregarding the "Shhhs!" from the people around us. I kept my hand on her hands to calm her and whispered to her to quiet down and wait for the intermission. I wondered if I should take her outside, but I was uncertain how to do that unobtrusively in the middle of arias and choruses. I knew how much she loved the music and what a special occasion this was for her. But the people in the row in front started whispering complaints. One of the men turned around quickly, squeezed my hand hard, and angrily hissed, "Hush her up!"

Fortunately, we made it through to the intermission without further incident. I was sweating and panicked, but I could see in Joan's face how thrilled she was by Verdi's glorious music. I tried to explain to the people who had complained that my wife had dementia and that I was doing my best. "Dementia!" they said, *laughing.* "Get her out of here. She shouldn't be here." Their rudeness and lack of sympathy made me want to tell them off, but I felt conflicted. They were cruel but probably right, I realized sadly. I shouldn't have exposed her, or anyone else, to this. And yet her face was so alive with enjoyment, I wanted her to hear the most beautiful singing, which was yet to come. Didn't she deserve some happiness in the midst of the horror of her disease? We stayed, and somehow got through the whole opera, which was magnificent, but I spent most of my time holding her hand and reassuring her, expecting at any moment that she would lose it and break down. As the applause flooded the hall, I looked at

Joan, who looked back at me with a smile and tears in her eyes, saying, "Wasn't that wonderful!" Relief mixed with happiness and a feeling we had just made it. But the sense of what if . . . ? made me smile back, kiss her cheek, and, arm firmly in arm, take her outside as speedily as the surging crowd would permit us to exit.

On several occasions, Joan seemed to be happy, only to explode with anger at Sheilah or me because of some inner dialogue she was having with voices representing people from our past, or shadowy figures her disordered mind had conjured out of thin air. Each time, in a fury, she hit out at Sheilah or me with her hands. Yet ten or fifteen minutes later, she was smiling again and could not remember trying to strike us. Almost all the time, Joan appeared to know who we were, and also knew her children and grandchildren. But for about half a year before she was hospitalized, she would on occasion misidentify or not recognize some or all of us. It was not always clear that she didn't recognize us, because she would act as if she were confused and uncertain. Needless to say, everyone in the family found this troubling, but not nearly as troubling as the times she fell into agitation and aggression. In the vastly expanding literature on dementia, much has been made of the tragedy created by the loss of the most personal of memories, including those of loved ones. And I, too, found this a terrible reality. Yet for me, the explosions of anger and frustration directed at me felt much more troubling and were harder to deal with than Joan's loss of memory. That I was now reduced to wondering which of these two terrible options was preferable shows just how bad our situation had become. Nonetheless, there were still days that were uneventful, which tended to mask the reality of how bad Joan's condition was by now. They served to prolong my state of self-serving denial that we were rapidly approaching a watershed. I simply wasn't prepared to see things as they were.

During this period, I was able to take advantage of a well-earned sabbatical. Friends in China urged me to bring Joan to Shanghai, where I had a collaborative research project that had stalled. They impressed on me that a network of friends there would be available to care for her and that, if anything, the care-giving would be better for her and for me there than it was here. As I was considering that option, another friend in the Nether-lands arranged a distinguished visiting professorship there later in the academic year. Joan was excited about both opportunities, but I worried about whether we could actually make these trips. Could I get her there and back safely? What would it be like to live abroad with her Alzheimer's? We sought the advice of family, friends, and doctors, and we ended up deciding to travel. We would fly to Shanghai via Taipei and Hong Kong. The short visit to Taiwan would be Joan's farewell to friends and colleagues whom we first met in 1969. It would also be a celebration of nearly four decades of research on things Chinese.

While we waited for our flight in a business-class lounge in Los Angeles Airport, I went to the bar to get us cups of coffee. When I returned, I found chaos. Frightened by my absence, and uncertain where I was and where she was, Joan had gotten up and walked into the sharp edge of a glass coffee table, opening up a deep laceration in her lower leg. Blood was everywhere. The at-tendants tried to help me clean and bandage the wound. We just made our flight, but for the next month in Taipei and Shanghai the wound required constant attention: medical visits, minor sur-geries, and twice daily cleaning and bandaging. I did everything that was asked of me, but I felt for certain that I was now at my limit. Fortunately, our Chinese friends rotated assistance with caring for Joan, just as Anne and Peter and others had done, picking me up off the floor when I had reached my limit in Cambridge. The support our friends in Shanghai provided was so substantial, effective, and warmly human—and thankfully well received by Joan (who could still understand some Chinese)—that the stay there proved to be, as my Chinese colleagues had predicted, something of a respite, an easier time than when we were at home. To me, this reflected both the impressive responsiveness of Chinese social networks to members with health problems and the love our colleagues had for Joan.

Our entire family came to join us in Amsterdam, where we stayed at a charming hotel on one of the inner canals. Three times each week, Joan and I took the train to and from Leiden, where I was delivering lectures. On one trip, as we disembarked, Joan began to fall between the train and the platform, but I had by then developed the habit of keeping a very close eye on her and was able to catch her in time. I was shaken, but Joan didn't register what had happened. The next day was more terrible yet. Joan woke up in the morning and, for the first time, failed to recognize me. I knew this could happen, but I was unprepared to deal with it. Terrified by what she believed was a strange man in her bed, she screamed and started hitting me. For well over an hour, I kept explaining as softly and gently but compellingly as I could that I was Arthur her husband, but she wouldn't believe me. She agreed to sit at breakfast with our son, whom she recognized, but she would not let me anywhere near her. She was convinced that I was some impostor whom she couldn't trust. Over the course of the day, Joan improved, to the point where she even laughed off the misadventure. But I was shattered. It's easy to say that her memory loss wouldn't interfere with my love for her, but quite another when she suddenly treated me like a stranger, with terrified, paranoid distrust. I understood what was happening medically, but existentially, it was as if the bond between us, strengthened into steel over half a century, could be snapped in an instant.

When we returned to Cambridge, Joan had a few more of those episodes. Sometimes she again became frankly paranoid, believing I was a stranger who had replaced her husband and was out to kill her. Each devastating episode revealed the depth of her fear, but she didn't talk about them afterward, or perhaps even remember them. I was left feeling isolated and vertiginous, as if I, too, were tumbling into the abyss that Joan occupied. As a psychiatrist, I could appreciate the experience of delusions for patients, and knew about Capgras syndrome, in which people suffer the delusion that someone close to them is an impostor, but I had rarely thought about their impact on family members. I was now sensitive to their experience on a deep, personal level.

Joan continued to unravel. She became incontinent of urine and had to wear adult diapers. On three occasions, she was fecally incontinent and defecated on the floor. I cleaned up the mess, washed the floor, and cried uncontrollably, sure that I couldn't go on any longer. Joan consoled me and cheered me on, as she had from the start: "You can do it! Arthur, you can do it," she implored. So I did it, and much, much more.

My clinical research experience has taught me that different symptoms and behavioral problems can carry greatly different meanings for different caregivers. For some, fecal incontinence is less upsetting than other conditions. But Joan had always been so elegant, controlled, and private in intimate matters that this consequence of her disease was especially difficult for me. It probably also reflected my own discomfort with bowel control issues—after all I was a psychiatrist, not a gastrointestinal physician.

Other family caregivers have shared with me similar experiences of feeling paralyzed by their loved one's decline into a low level of self-control and functioning. To many, it represented a wall they simply could not climb, until their disabled family member insisted, as Joan had, that they could do it, make it over the wall. And, to their surprise, they did just that. They pushed on. This is what I mean when I talk about care recipients playing an active role in the reciprocity at the heart of caregiving even in the direst of conditions. Here it was Joan who gave me the wherewithal to keep going.

In the summer of 2010, we were going through a very bad few weeks. Joan was nearly constantly agitated, even after taking a variety of psychoactive medications. Every other day she became violent: screaming, hitting out, delirious. Finally, on July 4, I decided we needed to get away, and Joan agreed. I drove three and a half hours to our vacation home in Maine, which we had not visited since fall. I settled Joan in a comfortable armchair, unpacked, keeping up all the time a running account of how the water looked, the color of the sky and the land, the beauty of the tall fir trees and fractured rocks. Eventually I fired up the grill. This being Independence Day, I barbecued hot dogs and hamburgers, corn on the cob, and tomatoes. In the kitchen I heated up a pot of baked beans. As we ate on our deck, we were overlooking the deceptively calm Damariscotta River, which is in fact an estuary of the Gulf of Maine and carries the unpredictable force of the sea. Just as the wind, swells, and waves can pick up quickly and turn a pleasant summer day into a sudden storm, Joan's emotional state changed rapidly for the worse.

Before I knew it, she was shaking with fear, panic, and confusion. She no longer knew where she was or why I had brought her here. I had developed a sixth sense that warned me when she descended into near delirium. It told me now that I had to take her home before she broke down completely. My stomach tightened and my heart started to pound as I packed everything up and shut down the house. I kept talking to Joan to make things seem right. But they weren't right; they were terribly wrong. We got into the car. Joan started fidgeting with the door handle on her side of the car, undoing the lock. Fearing she would open the door while I was driving, I held both her hands in her lap with my right hand, while I drove with my left for another three and a half hours, deep into the night. When we arrived back at our Cambridge home, I was exhausted and at my wits' end.

Back in our house, Joan went wild, thrashing about violently, smashing framed photos and several antique plates. She became acutely paranoid and shouted that I was a stranger who planned to hurt her. She lay on the floor kicking and screaming. I had done all I could, and it was not enough. Feeling helpless, I slumped to the floor, bereft of any cogent thoughts or words. Even tears wouldn't come. I felt utterly useless, unable to imagine any way to make things better. I didn't see how I could go on. I had reached a wall that I could not climb. I couldn't conceive of any way to alleviate the havoc and desperation that engulfed Joan, or the draining, crushing sense of abject failure.

When I share this story with other caregivers for people with neurodegenerative diseases, they respond, almost invariably, with a sad but knowing sigh of recognition and kinship. I have heard so many versions of the same story about the moment they broke down or gave up—a cautionary tale of the limits of caregivers. And yet these stories of desperation all end the same way, with the caregivers, broken and empty, somehow getting themselves up off the floor and back to the work of care. When I think about neurologists, the professionals who deal every day with cognitive decline, I wonder if for some it might be the fear of having to confront this profoundly disturbing mixture of defeat and hopelessness, even if transiently, that keeps them so tight-lipped and seemingly insensitive to the demands of caring for such patients.

Later that Fourth of July night, when Joan, who was still on the floor, finally fell asleep, I got up and called a colleague for advice. She recommended that she bring over a friend of hers who was an expert on psychiatric medication for patients suffering advanced dementia. They came that same night, and together they spoke with Joan, who had awoken, thankfully, without the delirium, although still extremely anxious and frightened. Taking me aside, they recommended that she be admitted immediately to a geriatric wing of McLean Hospital. There, they advised, her condition could be better assessed and a more effective regimen of antipsychotic medications developed that would control her agitation and delirium.

At the same time, however, they told me that the time had come for me to seriously consider placing Joan in a nursing home that specialized in dementia care. I didn't sleep that night. In bed, beside my wife, I felt defeated. I went over in my mind how months earlier, Anne, Peter, and I had looked at assisted-living and nursing home options for when Joan's condition would be too much for me to manage, and had come away shaken by the experience because most of the places we visited were unacceptable. I had known this was an inevitability, but my own denial, after nearly a decade of catastrophes, had been so fierce that I thought we were still months away from having to make this terrible decision. Now we were headed toward it at what felt like warp speed.

Why is this decision so extraordinarily hard to make? Why do we resist accepting it as the only viable way of going forward? I remember feeling this way after the director of an excellent assisted-living program in a leafy Boston suburb told me that in her opinion I had kept Joan at home too long. The director believed that at the time we were considering her impressive facility, Joan was already too impaired to be in assisted living and required, instead, a nursing home–level facility to care for her. Of course, I was annoyed by her admonition, which seemed to presume that this expert had the right to decide what was too long or too short a time in home care. But now, on reconsideration, it was clearer to me that there were alternatives, like assisted living, which I had for years not allowed myself to consider.

I had treated home care as the only choice for as long as I could sustain it. The last year or eighteen months had been hell for me and for Joan. Looking back, I could see that we had barely survived that horrible time. I don't know if assisted living should have been an earlier alternative, but a cognitive care unit surely would have been appropriate if I had made the decision that home care was no longer possible.

I had been mule-like in my stubbornness. I was going to take care of Joan at home no matter what happened. I had promised her, and she expected me to keep that promise. It was as simple as that. But, of course, it wasn't so simple. The woman to whom I had made that promise was not the same woman after almost ten years of destructive dementia. Nor was I the same caregiver. I was exhausted, physically and mentally. And Joan? Well, that was the problem, wasn't it? I could not accept that the Joan I loved and felt indebted to had gone, was no more.

I could not accept this line of reasoning, because my own commitment was not rational. It was absolute, not relative. And though it was based in love, it was also sustained by guilt. I am certain I could not have said this at the time, because I could not see it, or rather I wouldn't allow myself to understand it as such. That guilt was embedded deep within me. I had for thirty-six years been sustained by Joan's care. She had never given up on me, in spite of the immense burden I had placed on her. How could I give up on her after only ten years and still face myself in the mirror? Or face my children? Or my mother and brother?

Anne and Peter had recognized that something had to be done differently, long before I reluctantly escorted Joan to McLean Hospital. They saw that I was at my limit. They understood that Joan had to go into a nursing home, and had gone with me to look into the options. So why my mulish persistence? In one sense, it was the inertia built up in the very habit of doing the work of caregiving that resisted change. At the end, I knew deep within that I could not keep going, but I kept going anyway. In another sense, it was the irrational fear of failure. I had in my lifetime persisted in everything; it was my strength, and my nemesis. I did not give up. I did not allow myself to quit. I acted as if I could never be defeated if I forced myself to keep going—no matter the personal price I paid, or that others had to pay.

Guilt was there, of course, long before Joan. It went back to my early brutal life. Unconsciously, I suppose, it went all the way back to an absent father. Had I driven him away? Had I not been worthy of his love? These are not rational thoughts. But the unconscious is not rational. Caregiving for me, at its deepest, was redemptive. It redeemed me. Didn't my mother say it made me human, meaning that until then, I had been somehow less than human? All of these intrapsychic meanderings came crashing down on me when I allowed myself, as an act of self-preservation, to give up on caring for Joan at home.

Of course, this picture could be played back in reverse, from Joan's situation with me as the peripheral figure. Her condition had deteriorated to such a point that no matter what I and my family felt, a nursing home was all that was left as a choice. The alternative was now unsustainable. It had come to an end. I would continue to be part of the caregiving but no longer in the central role. From this point onward, I was as much an observer as a participant. Many others have struggled for the words that describe this tragic transformation. However it is expressed, it is about caring at a distance mediated by an institution and its staff. We had arrived at long last at this final place.

And so we came to what would turn out to be the final nine months of a long and grueling journey. The end of the course of the Alzheimer's disease. The end of Joan Kleinman.

Ten

W ell before Joan's illness had reached this crisis, you will recall, Anne and Peter had helped me to look into a nursing home that specialized in dementia. We visited over two dozen such programs in and around Boston and discovered an enormous disparity in the quality of facilities, staff, and activities. One such unit in a nearby small private hospital was downright appalling: patients were lined up in wheelchairs near the elevators on each floor, unkempt, soiled, flailing their arms to call for assistance that clearly was not forthcoming. Other facilities were only marginally better; visiting them was depressing. On the other hand, we also found several heartwarmingly impressive institutions, not necessarily the most modern but with dedicated, caring staff and remarkable programs.

It must be acknowledged that compared with most other families, we came into this process with a multitude of advantages. We possessed the financial resources, the time, the connection with the health care system, and the medical knowledge (another kind of resource) not only to make an informed decision about where to place Joan but also to be able to secure a spot for her. I despair to think how difficult it must be for people in similar straits who lack such resources. Caregiving generates so much anxiety and unhappiness, and the search for an institutional placement is one of the more dispiriting and challenging aspects of the experience.

Several nursing homes turned us off immediately, simply because of their grim architecture, cramped quarters, limited staffing, or sometimes just a pervasive background smell of urine. These superficial features can tell a lot but can also mask more significant truths about the qualities of the facility. I remember the day when Peter, Anne, and I pulled up in the rain-soaked parking lot of what seemed to be an unpromising nursing home. The outside was bleak and institutional. The carpet in the entrance hallway was old and faded, as was the flowered wallpaper. We entered a very small office off a dayroom that, while cheerfully arranged, was just as cramped. Unlike the other nursing homes we had visited, however, in this one we saw residents smiling, taking part in activities—singing, doing exercises, playing bingo and other games—and surrounded by lively and engaged staff. We heard laughter and conversation, and we saw people moving around. Someone had selected interesting background music and also taken care to put out a lovely flower arrangement. Even those patients who were limited to their beds had bright, clean, and airy rooms; they were attended to by obviously caring nurse's aides. The patients appeared to be treated with respect and kindness, so much so that a number of them smiled at us warmly as we passed their rooms.

The cramped dayroom was cheerfully arranged with frail elders, nicely dressed, in wheelchairs at tables that had been carefully set for lunch. In the tiny office next door, we met the unit's director: a very warm but no-nonsense middle-aged woman who had devoted her career and her life to dementia care. Unlike the professionals we had met earlier that day, who had left us feeling disillusioned and unsettled, this woman exuded excitement about her work and clearly communicated her aspiration to sustain a program that had earned an impressive reputation. In spite of the constraining conditions, she and her staff radiated a sense of purpose and genuine commitment to their demanding work. They spoke to us knowledgeably and with compassion about the details of the daily schedule. The director described the ethos we had already sensed intuitively in the dayroom and the hallways. She explained what made it special. We were surprised when we learned from others that her own mother had lived in the unit with end-stage Alzheimer's disease, but the director believed this was the best evidence of her commitment to this particular place as a special setting where care came first. She told us her leadership was moral more than managerial. Dementia care was her passion. Every staff member knew that and to one degree or another shared her motivation; indeed, they were selected and trained with this in mind. This remarkable professional caregiver had spent more than a decade in the confining space she and her colleagues had made so lovely, warm, and human. In the end, Anne, Peter, and I decided that in spite of our enthusiasm for the director and her commitment, the significant space and financial limitations were serious enough that we would look elsewhere for a nursing home where Joan would spend her final days. Yet we came away from our visit uplifted, much as other families surely did. What was it that made us feel entirely different than we had after earlier visits, even to one facility whose physical space was much more impressive and almost brand new? The milieu that this committed professional created was so obviously centered on the reciprocity between staff and residents, and on the presence of both. From the director to the aides and even the kitchen workers whom we met, the staff were driven by compassion, kindness, quality caring, and a clear moral vision of how people suffering from dementia and other disabilities could live in a real community. From an anthropological perspective, we could see the interactions as warm gift exchanges between people who had genuine human ties.

During our search for the right place, we met several directors of dementia units (all of whom were also women) who shared this woman's commitment. They were working under even more difficult and limiting physical and financial circumstances, with varying degrees of success. These individuals impressed us deeply, as did the staff of NewBridge on the Charles, the very fine cognitive care unit that we ultimately chose for Joan. Of course, we also met a number of less appealing characters. The worst of these had tripled up demented patients in formerly two-bed rooms like sardines in a can. He literally rubbed his hands in happy anticipation of what he told us would become a real business success. Others were simply mechanical in their care, or defensively tried to justify the disturbing conditions around them.

The really committed nursing home professionals seemed to regard themselves as occupying the ground between patients and their families, on the one side, and health care professionals, on the other, mediating between the two and offering services that were at the same time professional and yet part of family experience. They concerned themselves with relationships—with family and friends, professional consultants, the full range of staff members, and, of course, the residents of their facilities as a community—as much as with the disabled individuals in long-term care. These relationships brought families into a professional space and placed professionals and staff into family and friendship networks. Interestingly, the more impressive leaders of these units revealed that they came from families in which care for the elderly was a family tradition, that their parents and grandparents had performed the same work. In their families, they explained, the work was considered a moral calling, not just a business.

These committed professionals saw their work as part of a social network of family and friendship. They got to know their patients' families, in order to understand better the person they were looking after. A close friend told me a story about a woman who apparently had made her way out of such a facility. She was found sitting at a bus stop waiting for her long-dead husband to come home from work as she sometimes used to do, her family had explained. Realizing how fundamental this memory was for her, the manager had a garden seat and shelter erected in the garden where she could safely sit and wait. Another resident of such a care-oriented place would wake every morning before dawn agitated and fretful. In a family consultation, his relatives said he used to work scheduling train departures well before the rush hour at the rail yards. The staff were then able to reassure and calm him by telling him that the trains had all gone off on schedule and he could go back to sleep. I have come across other examples in the media as well that convince me that creating such a family-oriented atmosphere in an eldercare institution is feasible, if the value of caring is made central to the institution's mission.

These nursing home directors told me that they were a small part of a vast network of programs and activities that strengthened society and made the world a better place, but feared that these programs and activities would likely weaken and disappear without nurturing and attention. Some lamented that the human quality of caring, which they believed to be their calling, was being lost amid all the efforts at strengthening health care institutions. As one told us, "What isn't talked about enough, while we are talking about insurance and management issues, is how to keep doing caring at a high standard." These were rare individuals in a space suffused with suffering, where too many neglect or bully their charges and one another and an ethos of futility is commonplace.

The problems in caregiving we encountered with specialists, in the hospital setting and in searching for a nursing home, reveal ongoing challenges both in professional caregiving and in teaching care to students who will become the next generation of health professionals. Sadly, my family's experience is far from unique. Case after case illustrates why care is so constrained in health care facilities and in the broad system of health care that connects people with needs with bureaucracies, businesses, governmental agencies, and their cultures. A closer look at a few such experiences can help us identify some of the more pressing issues surrounding care.

One stands out vividly in my memory. On a slate-gray and bone-numbingly cold New England winter day in the late 1980s, I hustled down the street with one of my medical students to the hospital's outdoor parking lot. He stamped his feet to warm himself while I fumbled in my overloaded coat pocket to find the car keys. We thawed out as I drove to a patient's apartment in a working-class neighborhood. Mrs. Wilson, a large, seventy-nine-year-old Irish American widow, had adult-onset diabetes that her doctors regarded as under good control. However, peripheral vascular and cardiac complications had left her with complaints that seemed to her physicians out of proportion to the modest degree of pathology they had carefully documented. I had been asked to consult on the case because of the large discrepancy between the physicians' notes, which described minimal medical problems, and the patient's own severe complaints. The blood glucose readings were in the normal range, as were her other tests—electrocardiogram, X-rays, and measures of the circulation in her legs. Still, Mrs. Wilson complained that her condition was "terrible" and that she couldn't go on. The doctors labeled her a "difficult patient." The fact that she fairly frequently missed her appointments with them made matters that much worse.

After the case was presented this way to me, I had phoned Mrs. Wilson, and since she said she couldn't come to the clinic, I asked her permission to make a home visit together with the medical student on her case. She readily agreed. I recalled the home visits that had been so seminal during my own medical education, and that had first begun to open my eyes to the real meaning of care, and I knew this visit could have similar value to my student. I had often made home visits in my medical anthropology research, but rarely had I done so as a clinical psychiatrist and medical school teacher.

We arrived at an old, run-down triple-decker apartment building that seemed to have shriveled and contracted under the relentless cold, its paint flaking off, but the nearest parking spot we could find was three city blocks away. The student and I ran back to the building, arriving so numbed by the frozen air that we spent several minutes in the closed entryway trying to warm up before taking the two flights of stairs to her small apartment. Inside, we found Mrs. Wilson dressed in a heavy white wool sweater with mittens on her hands, seated in a large, heavy armchair, almost on top of a small electric heater, whose warmth did not reach us. We kept our coats and hats on because, impolite as I knew it was, we needed them for their warmth against a cold that seemed to penetrate right through the walls.

Mrs. Wilson explained that something was wrong with the boiler, which she suspected was the original in this century-old house. Apparently, the problem with the boiler also affected the water heater. No matter, her apartment was still warmer than the bitter cold outside. We learned that Mrs. Wilson got so cold when she went outside that she simply couldn't face up to walking the six blocks to the nearest food store. Hence, she informed us, her antique refrigerator was almost bare. She had called the grocer, whom she knew slightly, a week before, in order to have food delivered. But the heavy bags were left in the downstairs hallway, and she got short of breath carrying the bags up the two flights of stairs. She didn't believe she had the strength and stamina to do that again.

She was the widow of a Boston policeman whose family lived in Ireland. Mrs. Wilson's own family lived in the Midwest. She and her husband had no children, and her two best friends had died several years before. She had moved to her current apartment a year ago, because on her limited Social Security income and the small pension her husband had left her she could no longer afford the rising rent in her former apartment in a gentrifying neighborhood miles away. The move, she lamented, had been a mistake. She knew no one in her building or on her street. She was cut off from her church and from the hospital, the two critical institutions in her life. She was, as I remember her saying, "Alone. All alone."

The student and I stayed for half an hour or so. When we left, we decided to drive to the nearest store to buy her bread, peanut butter, and jam (which she told us was her favorite food), soup, vegetables, and fruit. The student ran up the stairs to deliver the bags of food, refusing the money she offered.

Back at the hospital, I asked him to write up the home visit in a medical-style note in Mrs. Wilson's chart. That report, I told him, should include our diagnosis of the social problems of isolation and her intolerable living conditions. It should make concrete recommendations about what urgently needed to be done for her, such as assistance from a social worker, an arrangement for getting delivery of Meals on Wheels, help getting to the hospital, alternative housing with attention to her functional limitations, contact with community groups, transportation to get her to her church, consultation with her family and Mrs. Wilson about the future, and so on.

Almost nothing that we reported had been known by her medical team. No one knew of her marginal financial state, her isolation and loneliness, or the extent to which she was compromised and disabled by her poor living conditions and especially the stairs she could barely climb. No referral had been made to a social worker to get her additional social assistance. And not one of her professional caregivers had had any idea at all what it was like in freezing winter weather for her to try to get to the hospital. The notes about the discrepancy between objective measures and subjective experience were created in almost total ignorance of what it was like for her to struggle with her limitations in the real world.

I was angry, frustrated, and nearly despondent at the appalling lack of progress. The lesson I had learned so many years before in medical school, about the social context of care, about human connections, apparently still hadn't been learned. I had devoted my career to bridging the divide between medicine as a technical and scientific practice, on the one hand, and the lives of real people in real families in real communities on the other, and yet here we were, after all that time, brought low by the stupid, lazy failure to ask a patient a couple of simple, meaningful questions. In that moment, I felt like something of a fraud, as if all the accolades and distinctions I had received as a champion of social medicine and the human element of care were now quietly mocking me. Deep down, I had believed that the efforts of so many teachers and thinkers and researchers and activists had brought about real change in the practice of care, so how could a case like this still baffle medical professionals, and how common were such cases?

The medical student shared my sense of outrage about this patient. This was a teaching moment, and I felt humbled seeing the revelations wash over the student as they had washed over me. At the same time, however, I felt that it wasn't only that student who needed the lesson, but also the entire medical staff, including me. All of us had lacked the empathetic imagination to ask her the kind of questions that would have revealed her precarious situation. As someone wholly responsible for her own care, she was desperately constrained. The professionals had failed her. They knew a lot about her disease pathology, but almost nothing about her experience of symptoms and disablement, or how that experience was shaped by the particular circumstances of her life. What they had mistakenly attributed to the exaggerated symptoms of a chronic complainer was in fact the stoical endurance of a brave woman.

Because her doctors and other clinical professionals had confined their gaze to a narrow spectrum of her experience—her pathology—neither her physicians nor the hospital's managers appreciated what she most needed. This failure is not confined to one Mrs. Wilson, but to so many who enter the health system lacking the funds, influence, knowledge, family, or friends to be their resources, agents, or advocates. It is long-standing and it is getting worse. Call it an absence of compassion or breakdown in caring, but see it for what it is: a fundamental question of which values matter most to health care professionals and which ethos of practice they are willing to accept. This is a human problem and it has a human solution.

In the early 2000s, I was asked by a local private health care system in Boston to develop a case-based teaching module for their clinical centers throughout the area. The goal was, first, to sensitize the staff in each center to how ethnic and cultural differences between patients and doctors create problems for caregiving, and second, to suggest ways to prevent or ameliorate those problems. Working together with an African American pediatrician-anthropologist, we interviewed patients whose care had been compromised by problems the staff regarded as principally cultural. One of the people interviewed was an immigrant Haitian mother who had missed a number of medical appointments for her five-year-old HIV-positive son. The surprising question put to us to guide our evaluation was whether to connect via satellite phone hookup with a practitioner of voodoo in Haiti to develop a culturally appropriate intervention.

The Haitian mother, we learned, was also HIV positive. She was an overworked nurse's aide who possessed a full understanding of AIDS and its treatment, including what was required of her in caring for her son. She wanted to provide him with the best care, and by and large succeeded in doing so, but a combination of work and financial constraints limited her ability to bring him to all his scheduled medical appointments. She worked the graveyard shift in a nursing home from 11:00 p.m. to 7:00 a.m. When she left work she immediately drove to her friend's apartment, where her son slept on her work nights. She took him home, bathed and dressed him, fed him a substantial breakfast, and assiduously made sure he took all his medicines. Then she drove him to a private day care center, where he stayed until 5:00 p.m. This barely gave her enough time to go shopping, clean the house, wash their clothes, prepare a meal, and go to sleep for five hours or so. After waking, she picked up her son at the day care center, served him dinner, played with him, got him ready for bed, and drove him to her friend's apartment, where he had his own room and could be watched over by an attentive caregiver. Following that, she returned home and paid bills, called friends and relatives, and did whatever else she was required to do to hold their lives together. At 10:30 p.m. sharp, no matter how sleep-deprived, stressed, and exhausted by her inhuman schedule, she drove to work. She missed appointments for her son only when they were for routine follow-up and she felt she had insufficient time and energy to drive him to the clinic. The parking fee, which was surprisingly high, was another deterrent.

At first, the clinic's nurses and doctors were annoyed with us for presenting this case as a set of social issues, and playing down the cultural elements, which were supposed to be our focus. When we responded that we didn't believe her Haitian culture was relevant, they seemed incredulous about the moving story that we reported and that no one in the clinic had previously elicited. The clinic's patronizing staff simply fell back on an exotic (and irrelevant) cultural stereotype, and wrongly accused the mother of noncompliance as a way of covering over their near-total ignorance of the brutal social reality of her life.

Readers may wonder how this could still be. How could this woman and her son attend a pediatric AIDS clinic for several years and yet have no one in the clinic understand the context of their lives? The endemic inattention in the health care system to the human stories behind illness flies in the face of what caregiving by professionals should be about. The failure of practical wisdom and emotional imagination among medical professionals is a kind of moral blindness. I call it a moral problem because such radically different values are at play for professional and family. Families, over the long trajectory of an illness, live in a daily world of hope, frustration, exhaustion, and caring work. They share the experience of the ill person's state and needs on the most intimate and specific level. Health professionals, by contrast, enter that experience only for brief, fragmented clinical moments, usually without context or meaning, unless they stop long enough to ask, and listen.

My own understanding of this phenomenon deepened through contact with family members of patients with Alzheimer's and other neurodegenerative diseases. Over the decade of Joan's downhill course, we met many patients and families in hospital waiting rooms and cafeterias. My articles on Joan's and my experiences also elicited numerous responses from family members and close friends of seriously impaired neurological patients who had undergone experiences much like ours. Almost all voiced similar concerns about the professional care they and their loved ones had received. They consistently described the practitioners on whom they relied as not only disappointing and unhelpful but also ill informed about and indifferent to what they, the family caregivers, experienced as the real challenges of caring for a seriously ill family member.

This gap was partially filled by social workers, community organizations, and nongovernmental organizations, but their resources and reach were limited. Many medical staff appeared uninvolved and uninterested. Those physicians, nurses, and members of other health care professions who showed concern and real interest in helping people cope were greatly valued but atypical. Each time I heard these complaints from families, I felt a rising defensiveness, because as a physician I felt threatened. And then my identity as a family caregiver would kick in, and I would find myself nodding in agreement. It was saddening to listen, but even more so to have to agree. Compounding my angst was the nagging sense of futility, knowing how far the greater medical community still needed to move to meet the unspoken desperation of carers for understanding, guidance, and support.

Yet there are hopeful signs. In recent years I've come across many clinicians who still struggle to advocate for their patients in the hospital, their consulting rooms, the management committee, over the telephone with insurers, at the computer terminal, and in the corridors and offices of health care bureaucracies. They persist despite all the hurdles: time pressures, workload, rules, financial arrangements, policies, and codes of practice. Above all, they have to work within a professional value system that limits the care they provide. This is true not only of physicians but also of the nurses, physical therapists, occupational therapists, and other types of professional caregivers who traditionally shoulder most hands-on caregiving in our health care system.

Most of us, at one time or another, have felt some kind of division within ourselves. This internal conflict may have been between material desire and ethical aspiration, remembering and forgetting, ambivalence and commitment, professional ideals and practical reality, or other values and practices. In caregiving, there is the common tug-of-war between the sometimes bitter feelings that care is a burden and the more heartening certainty that, no matter how burdensome, it is ultimately rewarding. Caregivers can experience these competing emotions at different times or at the same time; caregiving practices can feel simultaneously burdensome and enriching. But we cannot expect caregivers, who already bear such heavy responsibility, to simply dig deeper within themselves to find the strength to reconcile these inner conflicts, and so to resist the exhaustion, irritation, or resentful resignation that sometimes consume them. They need the support of health care systems that value and prioritize care and context, and so encourage that caring self to emerge and flourish. Put differently, although it may cost us something, we can acknowledge and enable the world of family care by humanizing professional care, ensuring that these professionals value what we as individuals are trying to accomplish.

Adele George was a lively, petite, gregarious southerner whom I had taught when she was an undergraduate and a medical student. She called me during her first year of residency at a Boston hospital to say she needed to talk with me. I could hear the tension and apprehension in her voice. When we finally found a mutually convenient time, she reported, in an uncharacteristically hesitant voice, an incident that had shaken her so much that she had started to question her postgraduate medical training and the stability of her own values. She reminded me that she had, from elementary school onward, always wanted to be a physician, a doctor who cared about patients and who valued above all else attending to their experiences of suffering. I hardly needed reminding; I had every confidence that Adele would do all she could to put her patients first.

The incident she described took place on a hot and humid summer night during the first year of her residency in internal medicine. She had already had an extremely busy day in the wards and, because of a mix-up in scheduling, she was also on call in the hospital that evening. There were emergency admissions and other serious clinical problems that had kept her up to 2:00 a.m. Less than a half hour after she had fallen into a deep sleep in the on-call room, she was awakened by the insistent ringing of the telephone. Adele was understandably exhausted and confused. The nurse on the line said that there were several patients who required her immediate attention. She pulled herself together and quickly made her way to the hospital room of the first patient on the list. There she found a middle-aged woman who was to undergo a major surgical procedure later that morning and whose intravenous line had become blocked. The nurse had been unable to get the IV restarted or put in a new one. Adele started a new IV and ran off to see the next patient on her list, so that she could get some sleep before early-morning rounds with the senior resident and attending physician.

As Adele made for the door, this woman told her in a shaky voice how frightened she was of the upcoming surgery and how much she needed to talk. Adele found herself responding almost automatically, "I'm sorry! I can't stop right now to talk to you. I have other patients to see." With that, she ran down the hallway. But after twenty yards or so she stopped, asking herself, "How could I have just done that? I went into medicine precisely because I want to listen to and speak with patients like this. And here I am running away." She turned around and returned to the patient's bedside, apologizing for running off, and spent the next half hour sitting on the bed, holding the patient's hand, and trying as best she could to answer her anxious questions about the imminent surgery.

By the time she finished with the other patients, there was no time to go back to sleep. Downing multiple cups of strong coffee, she prepared for attending rounds. After the rounds ended, when she could finally get out of the hospital and return to her apartment, Adele broke down, crying bitterly as she confronted the stark reality of her situation. Could she live up to her expectations of herself to be a caring physician and still survive the grueling residency? She knew from her education and reading precisely what was happening to her, and yet she still could not face the prospect that she would have to put aside what she valued most about medicine, just to get through her training. "If this is what it takes to make it," she said, "will I become a different person when I emerge from training: a doctor who has learned that the only way to resolve this desperate conflict between aspiration and practical reality is to cut corners to get the job done no matter how inadequate the human consequence for patients?" I spoke with her for more than an hour, pointing out that probably most of us faced with the same issue would have kept running down that hallway until we reached the next patient, and many would not have even thought twice about it. There was something in her that made her different and at least on this occasion, the person she wanted herself to be shone through in unmanageable circumstances. Still, neither of us was really satisfied by my response. We learn repeatedly that the forces that have aligned to prevent or discourage humanity in clinical encounters, attending to the messy realities of emotions and life circumstances, are truly powerful. The problem was a particular one, but a larger issue loomed. And neither Adele nor I had an adequate answer for it.

I have had a fair number of encounters with physicians and medical students that centered on this issue. One of the most disturbing was with a student who during the first two preclinical years as a medical student had demonstrated remarkable skills in interviewing patients. She had also carried out a small research study based in patients' social histories on the influence of social context on the course of chronic medical disorder.

In the initial week of her first specialty rotation in the clinical years (sometimes called the cynical years) of medical school, the junior resident asked her to take several patients' histories, record them on the chart, and then do all the scut work (look up lab reports, call consultants, track down other information, fill out forms, etc.) for several other patients. So interesting was the first patient's social history that she spent forty-five minutes in the patient's room. When she came out, the resident was furious, insisting that if she ever took so much time again "merely" taking the history, it would surely affect her grade for clinical work. He shouted at her to go and take the other histories as fast as possible, get her tasks done quickly, and not waste any more time.

Appalled, she looked for support from others on the clinical team, but no one seemed to agree that she had done the right thing. She had learned a stark lesson: she ran into the next patient's room, spoke quickly, listened only superficially, and wrote the history up as concisely as possible. She knew she was not learning what she should, nor using the history-taking as a way to build rapport and be an effective healer. This insightful young woman went on to say that she was sometimes ordered, as were the nurses, to administer various questionnaires aimed at scoring patients' pain, sadness, fatigue, and other symptoms. After filling out the questionnaire and speaking with patients to understand their answers, she came away with a real feeling for the patients' subjective state and the significance of their complaints, but all that was wanted from her was a statistic, a score that was recorded in the chart as a "fact." Whether the score was noticed or contemplated by anyone else was moot. But it was there—a disembodied number that satisfied a procedural requirement. No wonder so many trainees put up walls of cynicism and indifference to shield themselves from the encroaching dismay. More than the all-too-common depression and anxiety, their aspirations and convictions are under constant assault not just by the pressures of the clinical load but also by the dehumanizing expectations of the hospital routines and requirements. Survival in the hospital and in whatever outside life you can manage depends on learning how to work the system by cutting corners, spending as little time as you can get away with in human interactions that can be emotionally and morally taxing.

Complaints about professional care have become a common refrain, not just from patients, but from physicians as well. Here are a few examples of voices from research and clinical encounters I have had over the past decade that illustrate the problem.

A sixty-five-year-old man with worsening diabetes and associated kidney, visual, and metabolic problems described it this way: "They rush me in for a visit. There is hardly time to talk about what is happening. No one asks anymore how I am feeling. And then I am rushed out. I don't get a chance to tell all that has happened. Or even to ask about what is coming next. I am very angry and very disappointed. What good does it do?"

"You would think I was irrelevant to my disease from the way I get treated," said a thirty-nine-year-old college teacher with a chronic intestinal condition. "Nobody asks me about my ideas. When I make a suggestion, it's taken as if it came from left field. It makes me angry, and it makes me want to do something, anything really, to show them that I am part of this. Sometimes I purposely miss an appointment or don't comply with the treatment—as silly and futile as it is. I'm sore because I want to have my opinion respected, taken into account."

"I'm just so angry at them. They don't listen. I want to shake them by the scruff of the neck and tell 'em, 'Here, don't you disregard me.'" This sixty-four-year-old mechanic with chronic liver disease seemed about ready to give up. "What can you do? They make me so angry sometimes that I want to stop coming. Sometimes I don't show up. But it only makes things worse for me."

A middle-aged woman recounted this story: "My mother is ninety-three. She doesn't hear well. She needs someone to speak with her who can slowly explain what her dizziness is about and why it is so difficult to control. But the doctors and nurses don't even seem to have the time to speak to me so that I can explain to her what's happening. It's very frustrating. How can they use the word 'quality' to describe the care she gets? But there is no alternative."

"I was so scared that they would not give my dad all he requires," said a man whose eighty-one-year-old father was in a teaching hospital with stroke and heart disease. "They might write him off. Another eighty-year-old. Time to pull the plug. I read the papers, I know what doctors are doing to keep costs down, and to ration care. If you don't push 'em, you don't get what you should. Well, I pushed 'em for Dad. I simply don't trust people in the hospital. I watch what they are doing and I speak up."

The experience of health professionals is just as fraught. An experienced primary care physician in a managed care practice described it this way: "Something very deep and very bad has happened, is happening, to medicine. There is so little time, and so little emphasis on spending time with patients, talking to them, asking about their problems, explaining what needs to be done, responding to their fears and wants. It's all a new language: cost, efficiency, management talk. This isn't the language of clinical practice I was trained in. I feel frustrated and very, very alienated. I'm beginning to think it is not for me. I need to get out of it."

"We all know medicine is going through a revolution," explained another HMO-based primary care physician. "But you like to believe—have to believe—that the change offsets only the nonclinical aspect of care. But that's preposterous. So we can't even tell ourselves lies we can believe in. My institution doesn't seem to value any longer those things I was trained to believe are central to good care: a close, trusting relationship with your patients, good communicative skills, enough time to talk things over with patients who are going through bad times with their diseases, attention to what bothers them. That is not only the 'soft' side of care. You need to do these things because they really are essential. And if you don't, don't do them I mean, then what kind of doctor are you? What kind of care are you giving? It's really a moral issue. The managed care institution with all its paraphernalia has become more important than the patient. The relationship should be called 'patient-doctor-managed care provider,' because we spend most of our time on the management issues. I think that is a dangerous slide in the moral content of doctoring."

Last, and perhaps most worrisome, here's what a medical educator at a leading American medical school told me. "Sometimes I feel like a hypocrite. I am standing up before a room of medical students and teaching them things about communication and psychosocial skills in doctoring, and acting as if they have the time to do these things once they get into practice. They don't; they won't! They can't take the time, and they will not get the support they need from practice managers to do the things they know how to do and know they should do. So there we are. That is medical education today. Wouldn't you call that a pedagogic crisis? But for a medical educator is it also a moral crisis? What to do?"

For the sake of balance, it is important to recognize that, thankfully, many patients and doctors have a much more positive view of health care. Nonetheless, the disgruntled views I have shared here are supported today not only by a vast and growing literature from patients and family members, but by stories from professionals that run from the disappointed to the frankly cynical.

A close friend of mine, a physician near my age who is still in primary care practice, described his feelings and experience in a way that closely mirrors my own. "I would sum up my life as a physician this way: It is a great field with wonderful opportunity to do good for people in a highly practical way that really matters to them but also to learn a lot about life and about our greatly changing society. And yet there is a self-defeating effect to all the things our health care system gets wrong, from insurance to all the hospital and professional regulations. And that is a really big problem! A problem for us the providers, but also a problem, a big problem, for patients. I think the quality of care is not what it was in the past. And in future, I'm worried. Really worried! Medicine has so much potential to be great, to really help folks. But we are caught up in a mess right now [the health care system] and none of us knows what it will be like in future. So, there is some sadness in me as I approach retirement. The question is: How about the new generation of physicians? What will happen to them? Will they be there for their patients like me and you? Or will medicine become something different, altogether different for them and their patients? I mean disappointingly so."

One way to make sense of the threat to caregiving in medicine is to consider four seminal paradoxes that I have identified during my years of study. The first paradox is that traditionally medicine has defined caregiving as central to the practice of the doctor. Yet over the decades, caregiving has become increasingly peripheral to what physicians actually do. Neither sufficient time nor money nor attention is devoted to caregiving by medical institutions, and the work of the doctor has moved away from hands-on practice to high-technology diagnosis and treatment. Practice, furthermore, is mediated by electronic information that objectifies and dehumanizes patients and further distances them from their doctors. And yet doctors and health care institutions still insist caregiving is central to the practice of medicine. That's what I call a paradox.

The second related paradox is that the contribution medicine makes to the kind of caregiving described in this book is obviously relatively modest in comparison to what nurses, allied health professionals, and especially families contribute; yet the medical profession routinely disregards these essential partners. Physicians and health policy makers need to recognize and acknowledge either the diminished place of caregiving in medicine or the importance of the other areas where care is enacted. Wherever multidisciplinary teams and family-based consultation and decision making are the norm, there are demonstrable gains and benefits for all, but for those practices to flourish, practitioners need the time, permission, and proper encouragement to bring differing perspectives and resources to patient care.

The third paradox concerns medical education. Medical educators readily admit that they are unable to commit sufficient resources (money, faculty, time, and place in the curriculum) to implementing caregiving principles and practices. They also acknowledge studies that show that first-year medical students are more interested in, and better at, the practical and psychosocial aspects of care than graduating students are. This dispiriting finding suggests that there is something about medical education that actively disables students in caregiving, even as it equips them with so much scientific and technological knowledge. This invites a Swiftian "modest proposal."* Given this sad reality, why

---

* Jonathan Swift's essay *A Modest Proposal* satirically criticized lack of feeling for the poor in the midst of the terrible nineteenth-century famine in Ireland. In an attempt to create outrage among the English colonial masters for not doing enough to save the Irish people, he recommended that the Irish eat their children.

not drop caregiving entirely from medical school curricula? I've raised this idea with medical educators, but not one is prepared to consider it. Indeed, they reject the proposal out of hand, as if it were sacrilegious. Yet no medical school in the United States has taken steps to make caregiving the most central part of medical education. The cherished image of the doctor and his or her calling to heal and comfort, which often is what drew them into medicine many years before, endures in the face of overt contradictions.

The final paradox is that health systems reform and the revolution in medical technology—which were in part developed to strengthen caregiving by making diagnoses and treatment less prone to error and removing obstacles to providing better outcomes—have paradoxically weakened it. Most versions of the electronic medical record, for example, which is so useful otherwise, had, until recent changes, no place for nurse's notes or any other description of the day-to-day emotional and social condition of the patient. There is no logical reason why this should have been the case. Fixation on computer screens, furthermore, takes up more of the physician's time than listening and speaking to patients, and has become both a blessing and curse for doctors and patients alike. The surgeon and author Atul Gawande worries that the inevitable advancement of technology has "trapped a great many of us . . . all of us hunched over our screens, spending more time dealing with constraints on how to do our jobs and less time simply doing them. And the only choice we seem to have is to adapt to this reality or become crushed by it."* Research— some of it my own—has confirmed what our intuition tells us, that anything that detracts from the human interaction between

---

* Atul Gawande, "The Upgrade: Why Doctors Hate Their Computers," *New Yorker*, November 12, 2018.

ARTHUR KLEINMAN

physicians and patients diminishes the quality, and potentially the outcome, of care. Pharmacological advances create the idea of "miracle drugs" and transform the patient into a prototypical consumer of products who is more like a profit center than a lonely sufferer in need of human contact. The seductive advertisements on American television, prohibited in many other countries, for putative wonder drugs (with rapidly muttered warnings about the risks) highlights the obsession with the market for health care, for sales and profits. Health care becomes a transaction, rather than a relationship. You see this in psychiatry, where the ideal typical model is a physician with a prescription pad, not a wise psychotherapist. Parallels exist in virtually every medical subspecialty.

Physicians, to be sure, have ample opportunities to practice caregiving. When listening to the chest, palpating the abdomen, or taking the pulse, they can do so with a reassuring smile, a supportive touch, and words that build presence and hope. When doctors talk with patients about treatment and prognosis, they can listen carefully (looking away from the computer screen) and take time to explain procedures and medications clearly, including full and easy-to-understand responses to patient and family concerns. They can prepare family members and close friends for what to expect over the course of an illness—so that they (family and friends) can figure out how to create a network of practical support—before passing them off to a battery of social workers, physical therapists, and other staffers. They can foster the feeling that the patient's improvement really matters, as does the family's active engagement. The physician should use these and other practices to draw the patient and family into a useful, authentic collaboration and to establish themselves as healers, above all else. That alone may be enough to produce the useful biological changes that occur in the still-mysterious placebo response.

When I have presented these paradoxes at professional and academic meetings, they elicit knowing smiles from some and sighs of resignation from others. Sadly, they trigger defensive protests from those who stubbornly cling to an outmoded, romantic vision of the physician as a hero struggling successfully against the odds. Audience members often applaud me for waging the good fight in the face of what they describe as the overwhelmingly negative influence of the political economy, the institutional bureaucracy, and the transformative technology. Their laments are familiar: *"It is inevitable,"* they reason aloud, *"that care will be diminished and will become ever more constrained. This is because the very practical values of the working professional have been deformed, moving away from the primacy of care of the patient as a moral calling. Instead, the doctor is now viewed as an employee of big businesses in a marketplace of services who is expected to value cost over benefit, efficiency for its own sake, and standardized one-size-fits-all practice guidelines. This, not real quality, is what audits of doctors are about. Those audits from health care systems' managers,"* I am advised as audience members get hot under their collars, *"represent the bureaucratic indifference to clinical experience of an industrial business model that is about 'throughputs' and has lost sight of what doctoring should be about."*

Yet impressively, almost all of these sessions end, not with everyone lamenting an unsolvable problem but with people offering examples of successful local efforts to improve care and elevate its place in the training and life of practitioners. That is to say, almost everywhere I go, there are medical and nursing practitioners trying to improve or promote caregiving. They lead and inspire. They are the role models for the young physicians and nurses. A wave of small initiatives is building within medical schools, hospitals, and clinical practices. That wave includes selection of medical students based on evaluation of their empathy and interests in care as demonstrated in their family, school life, and community; examinations of students' interviewing skills; household visits to the disabled so students can gain an understanding of what home care entails; support groups for primary care practitioners focused on dealing with death and dying and other emotionally difficult subjects, including burnout; and hospital-wide efforts to train staff to attend more respectfully to patient and family requests, and to respond to the stress experienced by trainees. They include efforts to assist harried staff in focusing on how they affect and motivate others, and to raise their awareness about the potential harm—both to the ethos of an institution and to the performance of junior doctors and nurses—caused by bullying, humiliating, demeaning, or harassing others, even when those behaviors are unintentional and rooted in the high-pressure medical workplace. Conversely, they incorporate forms of professional recognition that send the message that kindness, mentoring, listening, and empathizing are the crux of the healing role. Sometimes all it takes is a culture where one is acknowledged simply for making a difference to a patient or a worried relative.

There are also new programs devoted to modeling patient care as collaborative, with an emphasis on patient education and family support. The cancer care team, the palliative care group, and the various members of narrative medicine and medical humanities programs demonstrate that quality care can be a practical goal. And then there are managers and clinical leaders for whom "management by walking about" is a mantra. Leaving the office or nurses' station and walking around a facility, talking with patients and families and staff at all levels, gains them a sense of the strengths and weaknesses, cares and convictions of those who do the work and those who receive the care. This is especially evident in the hospitals that have a clearly articulated mission and commitment, be they religious or secular, that are explicitly invoked and modeled at all levels of the organization. And this in turn requires leaders who embody these values and fight for their primacy among the attributes of the hospital's or nursing home's care providers, the recognition given exemplary staff, and the respectful regard for their colleagues and patients.

What keeps physicians struggling to do these small but critical things, I believe, comes out of the grain of clinical experience. Here the doing of care is realized in the elemental condition of being with, and having the authorization to help, another human being who is in trouble and acutely needs the reassurance and reality of assistance. How that value-laden encounter works its way out differs for each practitioner and student, but the possibility is there for revitalization of hands-on caregiving as a core professional goal.

Eleven

A nd so we came to the final nine months of what had been such a long and arduous journey, the end of Joan's suffering.

I think of this last period as a triptych of gathering and then complete darkness, followed by soft light rising. The first panel is our entrance into the belly of the great leviathan of institutional health care. Despite my connections and the fact that Joan's admission had supposedly been arranged in advance, simply getting her admitted took an entire day, beginning in the early morning in the emergency room of a Cambridge hospital from where she would be transferred ultimately to McLean. Slowly but progressively, over the course of that long day in the ER of waiting, waiting, and more waiting, Joan progressed from a manageable mental state through worsening levels of anxiety to outright agitation. She dissolved under the endless grind of the admissions process, a disastrous display of deadening institutional routine and bureaucratic indifference carried to an unimaginable extreme. Occasionally the inhumanity of it all was relieved by new human faces bearing the promise of some resolution, but as new staffers took over, they would express the same surprise—with exactly the same words and gestures—that we were still there and nothing was happening. I suppose they wanted to ease our obvious anxiety by getting us to laugh at a system that, like the sorcerer's apprentice, had gone wild, beyond anyone's understanding or control.

In the admissions unit at McLean Hospital, which we reached in the early evening, everything was repeated, not once, but four times: by attending, resident, fellow, and medical student. This included the same cognitive-status test with the same questions asked in the same way, again and again and again. The results were exactly the same with respect to Joan's level of cognitive functioning, but with respect to her emotions, they were worse on each successive test. In a moment of clarity, when the geriatric psychiatry fellow asked Joan to remember three objects that were the same ones asked by the others (brown coat, blue tie, and red apple), she shocked him by announcing she would not continue with such a "tedious" and "tiresome" test. He apologized, obviously thrown by her suddenly lucid and articulate outburst, saying that she was, of course, right and that he hoped if he were in her shoes he could respond so tellingly. That tiny, unexpected interchange was about the only moment of genuine humanity during the evaluation.

Finally, after three hours of our ordeal at the intake gates of McLean, Joan was admitted to the geriatric neuropsychiatry ward. Sheilah and I accompanied her there. It was 11:00 p.m., and the nurses asked us to leave the ward. I was suddenly consumed by a single, crazy thought: escaping from the ward with Joan and, in spite of her condition, taking her home. My whole being recoiled at the idea of leaving her alone in a psychiatric ward. Sheilah talked me out of this dangerous plan and was able to convince the nurses to allow her to stay in the ward with Joan until Joan fell asleep. Reassured, I kissed Joan goodbye and drove home. Shortly after getting home at midnight, I called Peter and Anne to recount all that had happened during that horrible day. When I got to the part about leaving Joan with Sheilah in the ward, I broke down and wept uncontrollably. I felt the most profound sense of failure, having promised Joan for years that she would always be taken care of at home. In the end, I just couldn't find a way to fulfill that promise. Nothing Peter or Anne said could calm me down or assuage the guilt I felt over a decision that was for me clinically necessary yet emotionally and morally unacceptable. In my dreams during the early-morning hours, I relived the vivid and unforgettable episodes of our life together, as if I could see the golden moments and the darker moments in a single long arc bending into the night.

Joan stayed at McLean for a week. During that time her condition stabilized enough on a new regimen of psychiatric medication to enable her transfer to a long-term cognitive care unit in the NewBridge on the Charles nursing home that Anne, Peter, and I had settled on, in Dedham, Massachusetts, about twelve miles from our home. We had been greatly impressed with the facility; it was new, well appointed, in a beautiful wooded setting of hundreds of acres of rolling hills and meadowland, and, most importantly, it had both an experienced and dedicated director and a staff who conveyed kindness, warmth, and humane nursing skills. I had to use all my professional connections to get her admitted there. Her new and last place of residence was a single room with a pleasing view that felt more like a hotel room than a hospital room. It was off a common kitchen area and dayroom and was flooded with light. Residents could always hear the quiet buzz of life going on, but they could also stay in the privacy of their rooms.

For a week after she arrived there, Joan was uncontrollable: thrashing, striking out, screaming, in a state of delirium that went beyond anything I had seen before. This darkening picture is still part of the first panel in the triptych. The unit's director reassured me that she had seen this kind of wild behavior before. It was as if, she calmly explained in the midst of the turmoil in Joan's room, people entering the final stage of dementia became aware this was going to be the end: the final way station on the road to death, and they fought against it with all they had left.

With Joan in such a state, I hired a friend of Sheilah's, and together, the two of them provided round-the-clock nursing for Joan that supplemented the care from nurse's aides. Soon, though, whether due to new medication or sheer exhaustion, Joan became quiet and tractable. Over the next several months, with distressing speed, she lost the use of her limbs, and she began sleeping for longer and longer periods. I visited every day, driving out from Cambridge while trying to continue my teaching, which helped me stay sane. I sat by her side and held her hand, kissing her cheeks and whispering in her ear, "It's Arthur. I'm here with you. Your Arthur." Sometimes she smiled in recognition and even repeated my name out loud, but more often she seemed lost in her own dying. I hovered between somber acceptance and passionate denial—it was all happening too quickly—and even though Anne and Peter and their families visited frequently, I felt lost, cut off from the world. Several family members of other terminal patients in the unit told me they felt the same way.

During those months, I was continually impressed with the attentive and compassionate care she received from the nurse's aides, most of whom were recent immigrants from Haiti. They had been nurses, social workers, and community health workers in both rural and urban settings there. Here in the Boston area, this was the only steady employment they could find, and despite the poor pay, they committed themselves to it fully. They were unfailingly kind, understanding, and careful with Joan throughout the six months of this penultimate stage of care. I thought back to the Haitian mother of the HIV-positive child and wondered if she could be on the night shift. She wasn't, but in the care given to Joan, I thought I saw the same attention she gave her son. Nurses came to check on her throughout the day, taking her vital signs and giving her medication.

Because this institution belonged to Boston's Hebrew Rehabilitation Center, there was a Jewish chaplain who checked in with our family on a regular basis. She heard Joan's story as told by each of our family members, since Joan was hardly communicating, and she listened to our stories about ourselves as well. Warm, thoughtful, and greatly supportive, she made clear that the unit would honor Joan's wishes about dying with dignity and without medical interference. Other members of the unit's caregiving team—a social worker, a psychologist, a psychiatrist, the hospice doctor and nurse, and, of course, the director—were there for Joan and supported our family throughout her time at NewBridge.

What repeatedly struck me—and Peter, Anne, and my mother as well—was the deep humanity of the care Joan and the other patients received at NewBridge. Even if semiconscious, residents of the cognitive care unit were wheeled into the sun-filled dayroom. Staff interacted with them frequently and actively. For those in earlier and less severe stages of dementia, there were games, films, TV, musical events, and plenty of family members about. Even the most severely disabled patients were included in the main social setting and never disregarded by the staff. Rather, they were engaged as if still present, and when things had to be done, like use of a lift to help residents go to the toilet, family members could participate. As it was for Joan, all the patients had uninterrupted access to nurses specially trained in dementia care, and to the other members of the care team, who modeled the best ideals of care. They were authentic. They acted as if empowered to make their own independent assessments of the level of care required and the quality of the care given, even as they carried out that work with so much humanity. The ethos they created was gentle and responsive. They purposefully opened space for each dementia patient—even those with serious disability—and family members to feel comfortable. I came away believing that Joan had received the best imaginable caregiving, and so had I. This stood in stark contrast to the dismal caregiving I had observed elsewhere during Joan's decade-long journey through the network of medical specialists at Boston hospitals. It confirmed for me that there's simply no way an institution can't provide humane and sophisticated long-term care if the leadership is thoroughly committed to this objective and both demonstrates and demands it. We had seen that vision realized in several of the facilities we looked into for Joan, and experienced it at NewBridge.

The middle panel of the triptych showed only complete darkness. It was the final two weeks. Joan had stopped eating and drinking. We, her close family members, sought to honor her long-repeated request, formalized in her living will and health care proxy, not to linger. It had become for us a sacred pledge. No intravenous fluids. No assisted respiration. No antibiotics. Nothing but her dying. Close friends came from Seattle, Paris, and New York to join Anne, Peter, their spouses, my mother, brother and sister-in-law, and our four small grandchildren: Gabriel, Kendall, Allegra, and Clayton, in a death vigil at the bedside. We told all the old memorialized stories; we looked at pictures from each stage of Joan's life; we began the caring for memories that continues to the present as I write these words seven years after the fact.

We collaborated on moistening her lips, putting small pieces of ice in her mouth to relieve the dryness, and rubbing skin cream on her face, arms, legs, and back. We massaged her muscles and combed her hair. We sang to her. We kissed her. We played music of a kind she had always enjoyed and that seemed appropriate at the end—harp, cello, piano. When she seemed in distress, we arranged for a morphine drip, and as her condition deteriorated we concurred with the hospice doctor's plan to increase the doses even if they further suppressed her respiration. We wanted this final phase to pass as quickly as it could so that she was not tortured by the dying. I hope she wasn't, but I'll never be able to know for sure. The morphine seemed to take away her struggle. The last hours had arrived; Joan appeared at peace; even though her breathing slowed, it wasn't labored. We drove home late at night that final day for a few hours of sleep. When the night-shift nurse called as she had promised, we rushed to Joan's bedside, but she had already passed on. We had said our goodbyes over the last few days. We felt relieved; the suffering was over.

Yellow, the color of the tightly drawn parched skin of her jaundiced and ravaged face. A strange resonance in dying that recalled for me the opening words of *The Thousand Character Classic*, the Chinese poem she had worked so hard to translate over more than a decade but had been forced to leave unfinished: "Azure and yellow are heaven and earth." It was as if she, carrying me along with her, was returning to the origin. Joan died on March 6, 2011, early in the black morning of a wet day. The snow was fast melting, and the melt was rushing through the grates in the street as if winter was flowing into early spring. The gravestone where her ashes are buried at Mount Auburn Cemetery, only two blocks from the home we had lived in since 1982, reads:

BEAUTY, WISDOM, GOODNESS
ABOVE ALL, LOVE

KLEINMAN

JOAN ANDREA 4 SEPTEMBER 1939–6 MARCH 2011

There is ample room for my name to be added when my ashes join hers.

The stone is made of South Dakota granite, a lovely rose gray. Her father's Swiss family had settled on a farm in South Dakota. White birch and maple trees frame the grave, with one huge, old, hard-worn American maple only a few feet away. Nearby is a pond whose green waters are crowned by trees with colors that are deep green in summer and red and burnished brown in fall. The grave is near a quiet residential street, so it feels part of the ongoing drama of life. In springtime there are flowers everywhere. But I think I find winter the most resonant time to visit. Leafless trees, cold snow covering the ground, ice on the pond, the day ending in late afternoon with the last long rays of sunlight passing into the advancing blackness—all seem to symbolize that horrific decade.

When we visit we adhere to the Chinese tradition of sweeping her gravestone of fallen leaves and dead branches, clods of earth, and dried flowers. The hallowed act of sweeping away and cleaning is itself for us a conscious continuation of our caring for Joan, to soothe and honor the ever-present ancestral spirit.

Joan's funeral commenced with a memorial service at the chapel at Mount Auburn Cemetery. It constitutes the third panel of the triptych. Many, many friends, family members, colleagues, students, and neighbors attended. The ecumenical service was organized and presided over by a dear friend and academic colleague who also happens to be a Protestant minister. We were still numbed with grief and consumed by all the primordial feelings that attend the death of a loved one. So our friend stepped in and helped us to think through what kind of ceremony would best honor the person Joan had been, what her life stood for, and how we wished to memorialize her. Together we selected the flowers, the music, the form and pace of the ritual, the spoken remembrances, the readings, and the actual burial of her ashes. The service was framed by the care Joan had taken in shaping her life and our family, by the caregiving she had animated, and by the care she had received. Each of the speakers turned to personal reminiscences of Joan, as if offering a square of fabric to be sewn into the great quilt of our collective memory. As at a Chinese funeral, a large framed picture of Joan with a black ribbon stood at the front of the pews, facing the assembly. We all bowed before it as we went forward to speak.

When the memorial service concluded and we set out to bring her ashes to the grave, there was a soft light in the sky. It brightened as the funeral procession advanced. We emphasized that, again as in a Chinese funeral, we were transforming Joan into a revered ancestor, one who should, through our reverence for her, radiate health, efficacy, and good fortune to the family. The explicit message was that she would remain an active presence in our lives and we would work to keep our memories of her alive. Transformed, to be sure, but still there. A source of light, scattering the darkness. Within the "painted windows and the storied walls"* of our psyches, we would, with care, arrange and rearrange the remembered vignettes, the catalog of images, and the

---

* Robert Louis Stevenson, "The Lantern-Bearers" in *Across the Plains, with Other Memories and Essays*. New York: C. Scribner's Sons, 1903.

intimate feelings so that Joan would continue to influence us as a moral exemplar. An exemplar of how to live a life and how to build a family in all its forms. By sharing memories and collectively stewarding them in what might be thought of as our family's archive, we would continue to care for Joan Kleinman, so that she would openly and reciprocally continue to care for us.

We divided her ashes into four unequal amounts. About half went into her grave. The remainder we shared: near our house on the Maine coast, I poured some over a boulder in the woods that Joan had named "the ancestors' rock" to commemorate her parents; some I took to China and placed secretly in a beautiful site in Changsha, where our collaborative research began. The rest I have kept in the study of our Cambridge home. I feel better knowing that her remains are still with me. Peter buried his portion on his farm in central Pennsylvania between woods and fields looking out over rising land and low ridges, under a memorial rock; a Chinese *feng shui* expert would approve. Anne has kept her portion in a library fireplace. (Books and hearth represent for her what her mother was about.) She endowed a linden tree in Central Park and a memorial plaque on the Literary Walk in the park. She also planted a flowering laurel bush near an old farmhouse she and her husband and our closest French friends own in Provence. And together we spread ashes and slipped Joan's Harvard ID with her picture behind the name card of a great chestnut tree in the Jardin du Luxembourg in Paris near statues of a stag protecting its family and a fiercely proud lion in a quiet corner near the back of the gardens, where when we were young we picnicked and where Joan had brought our children and grandchildren. Protective and fierce are adjectives that describe the quality of Joan's love for our family. (Not surprisingly, with the years, her ID has disappeared.)

Each year we try to visit her grave as a full family, either on the date of her death or on a public holiday. But we also visit frequently as individuals or in small family groups. After sweeping the gravestone, each of us reports to our family ancestor on what has happened over the previous year. Sometimes one of my grandchildren plays the violin or guitar and sings, and we all cry because we have managed to conjure up the sadness of her passing and of the transience of life. But like so many families, we end up smiling and laughing with funny remembrances and happy feelings for being together. Life goes on, and on. Not a bad way to commemorate the mutability and the continuity of a small human band moving through time; becoming more human through the actions of a lifetime, the centrality of relationships, and the art of living as a means of seeking order and beauty and goodness out of experience. In short, we care for our individual selves, one another, and our small world. I think Joan would be proud.

So many people, from every corner of society, find themselves thrust into the role of caregiver. It may begin with one person caring for another, but it rarely exists in a vacuum. Care—a process that requires presence, openness, listening, doing, enduring, and the cherishing of people and memories—ripples out to family and friends, colleagues and communities. The bittersweet exercise of so many deeply human qualities echoes through generations. It is an invisible glue that holds society together. Countering the forces of division and destruction that are also core to our human way of being, caregiving does good in the world. And doing good in the crucible of struggle and suffering and thwarted aspiration we experience as the real world is about all we can hope for to ease our collective way forward. Life is dangerous and uncertain enough to unsettle the most balanced of us, and all of us need care—not only from and for others, but for ourselves—to get through.

Seen this way, care is what makes it feasible for us to become social beings and to sustain and strengthen our collective existence. So how is it that we so routinely overlook it? What steps can we reasonably take to strengthen and improve it? When political and economic forces, the crush of bureaucratic procedure, and the daily encroachment of technology appear to be driving caregiving out of hospitals and communities, what can we do to sustain care?

Perhaps we begin best by recognizing that our assumption that caregiving exists permanently as a natural element in the human universe is superficial and unfounded. Care can atrophy and weaken when it is inadequately nourished.

The United States, for example, has gone through what pundits call a national debate on health care, with hardly any mention of the nature or worth of caring. We have talked endlessly about the finances, politics, and systems of health care as they affect insurance and medical treatment, without asking deeper questions about the care they are meant to provide. Our understanding of quality and measurement of outcomes fails to incorporate those dimensions of human experience that are what caregiving is about. We talk about controlling costs, cutting services, limiting benefits yet assuring access without specifying, access to *what?* We haven't established meaningful measures to evaluate care and its quality. We have failed to recognize, acknowledge, and properly compensate women for the huge contribution they make to caregiving. As a consequence, as more women enter the workforce and men continue to fail to replace them, there will be less domestic care. The contributions of minorities, immigrants, religious organizations, charities, and public services to care are neither well recognized nor sustained by adequate public resources. The number of home health aides is shrinking because the remuneration is so poor. These are among the most essential support services societies and individuals require to function. (Even the mortuary staff that attended to Joan's body turned out to be experts in caring for us while we grieved.) The problem, as some suggest, is not that we fail to quantify these experiences, but that they *cannot* be quantified, because they are essential human interactions, the soul of what health care is.

Because caregiving shines a light on human conditions as inescapably interpersonal—"Life is with people" as the old Yiddish aphorism goes—it stands in absolute opposition to the radical libertarian model that has become so popular and influential in our times. The every-man-for-himself mentality, which reveres the rights and needs of individuals more than concern for the greater societal good, is fundamentally wrong and out of keeping with how societies really work and how people live their lives. It creates an impoverished and dangerously warped value orientation. In contrast, a caring perspective changes how we think of governance, economic relationships, and security. Governance, seen through this lens, becomes not just the application of power or the establishment of social control, but the exercise of social care and the cultivation of caring individuals and communities. Presence, focus, selfless engagement, and mutual support would become instrumental to how we are governed.

Economic priorities, in an environment of care, must move beyond maximizing profits, productivity, and growth. There is also economic value in sustaining and strengthening carers and the relationships and institutions that support them. Institutions, founded in this mode, would value caring as much as they would value efficiency, diminishing the slavish commitment to metrics that foster bureaucratic indifference to human concerns. Bureaucrats would be empowered to make fostering human welfare an ethical priority. The security state also needs to be rethought from this alternative perspective. Its huge population of prisoners, its enormous expenditure on surveillance, and its obsession with prevention and protection, caricatured in its attachment to the right to own and use firearms, would be balanced by its commitment to securing and protecting care as one of its main functions. Then the breakdown in caregiving in families, communities, and professions would become a central security concern, while much of the apparatus of security today—from prisons to government spying on the public to the pervasive us-against-them survivalist mentality—would no longer be viewed as a righteous path forward but for what it really is: a grave threat to the social bond that holds us together. Does this vision sound too idealistic, too radical to ever come into existence? Perhaps, but why can't we take the first steps toward that goal? Even the most politically conservative among us, that element of society that likes to invoke the romanticized ideal of traditional, small-town values of self-reliance and neighborly cooperation, must recognize the practical social logic and political wisdom of a society that simply values care for the other, including social care, as the core practice that enables our communities to thrive.

As a society, we remain blind to the fact that care is everywhere, and I fear that this blindness results from a willful, although perhaps subconscious, self-deception. Care infuses so many everyday human interactions, in our schools, communities, religious institutions, youth programs, volunteer organizations, and countless other endeavors, to say nothing of the families and friends across the country who have given themselves to the daily care of a sick or disabled person. Perhaps it's useful to remain oblivious to this caring ethic in order to cling to the idealized image of the individual in society as a self-interested, autonomous agent. To recognize the centrality of care would be to shatter so many politically useful fictions: the self-made man, the self-sufficient pioneer, the rebel innovator, the superhero, the free agent unfettered by government, none of whom could actually exist outside the context of human interdependence. We ignore the practice of care in order to instill blind confidence and promote heroic independent action.

Such denial blinds us further to one bit of wisdom that Joan had forever internalized: care is about doing good in the world, and that doing good for others is a way of doing good for ourselves. It is an existential imperative to support the human condition. There's nothing new about this idea. Nor is it idealistic or romantic. It is the most sober and serious understanding of the human enterprise. In the light of this book's account of a journey of caring, it is as necessary for the environment and the community as it is for the body and soul of each one of us.

How would our world look if we were to enact this moral mandate of doing good through caring? Everything changes when we start out from this premise. How do we build this vision into our aesthetic, emotional, and moral education, and on a more practical level, into our policies and programs? Is it possible to imagine society and the state reorganized explicitly so as to advance care and maximize acts of humanity that advance community well-being? What would happen even in the business world if care—for all stakeholders, and for the communities that they serve, and in which they operate—was elevated to the status of profits? How would foreign affairs be negotiated? What would domestic justice look like? What of human rights, global health, environmental protection, or security of income and food? I know that in the anti-care political atmosphere of the United States today, this vision is likely to be dismissed out of hand as wholly naive and impractical. But why can't we imagine a future world where a different atmosphere opens a space for even a small change in our moral orientation? In other words, once we accept care as foundational to social life, and once we come to see caring activities that do good for others in the world as the wisdom of living, why can't we begin to organize policies and programs and even everyday attitudes and actions to remake our world? There are no historical or anthropological precedents on a societal level, as far as I am aware, so such change is radical, and thus unlikely. Yet in the broad sense, isn't this objective a logical conclusion to our investigation of caregiving? And as such, shouldn't we be exploring ways to bring it about via a moral movement for care? If not now, as in other troubled times, where risks to security, well-being, and peace abound, when do we seek to enact these values?

Anne-Marie Slaughter, who has written so persuasively with regard to the care of children, speculates about what it would take to support care in the United States today, and reasons:

> To support care just as we support competition we will need some combination of the following: high quality and affordable child care and elder care; paid family and medical leave for women and men; a right to request part-time or flexible work; investment in early education comparable to our investment in elementary and secondary education; comprehensive job protection for pregnant workers; higher wages and training for paid caregivers; community support

structures to allow elders to live at home longer; and reform of elementary and secondary school schedules to meet the needs of a digital rather than an agricultural economy.[*]

She shows that a number of these proposals have actually garnered bipartisan support in the US government. To this list she also adds a human right to care, which she views as a logical development of the women's movement in America. I can support all of her policy prescriptions, but find especially attractive her claim for a right to care as a basic human right. This would encompass both a right to professional care and a right to care at home for the sick and the frail elderly. This would also include an equal right for women (and men) who provide so much of that care as unpaid benefactors of society to receive the compensation they deserve. This list can stand as the policy objectives of *The Soul of Care*, too, to which I would add: reform of health insurance to provide all Americans with universal long-term care insurance, whether via Medicare and Medicaid or some other program, elevation of the professional status and training of home health aides, and incentives to encourage caring by institutional service providers for all professionals.

I was in a close friend's house in Sydney, Australia, struggling to find the right words to begin this book, when I heard voices just beyond the screened front door. Peering out to the street, I saw a young man slumped awkwardly in an electric wheelchair; he appeared to be paralyzed. In the hot sun, beads of sweat fell from his

---

[*] Anne-Marie Slaughter. Chapter 11: "Citizens Who Care," in *Unfinished Business: Women Men Work Family*. New York: Random House (2015): 231–247.

contorted face. Behind him was a large SUV with its door open. At either side of his chair stood an elderly man and woman. The woman held a cup with a straw for him to sip from, while the elderly man wiped his face with a carefully folded towel. At the same time, the old man reassured the younger one in a brave and cheerful tone, which produced a crooked smile from his charge. Then the woman determinedly pushed the wheelchair up to the car's rear door, and they both struggled mightily to get their son (or more likely grandson) seated with a safety belt around him. I could see this effort was not easy for them or for him. In a few minutes, the car backed out of the parking place and they were gone.

There was a time in my life when I might have looked right past this scene without registering its significance. Yet on this day, contemplating writing the book I was already calling *The Soul of Care*, it held my attention completely. From experience, I could recognize the difficulty that's involved for all of us in the simple act of getting into or out of a car, and from there I could imagine the life of care led by this family. I recognized that brisk, upbeat tone of voice and knew how hard it might be to maintain while managing a demanding physical chore, like helping a spouse into a bathtub or a disabled grandson out of his wheelchair and safely into a seat in the car. I knew how simple tasks like those could occupy much of a day, and how accomplishing them could feel like an important victory. I knew the fear of letting a loved one down if the outing did not go well. I knew, even in this brief moment of witness, how much could be at stake. And I thought I also knew that this elderly couple, like me, had experienced the secular equivalent of the biblical appeal: Here I am. I am ready.

And so, at the end, the soul of care pivots to care of the soul. The active, direct doing of care—the caring in caregiving if you will—works on and through relationships to reshape the self. Drawing presence from deep within a caregiver and a care recipient creates a bond between emotion and meaning. That bond draws on the energies of the person, while at the same time reinvigorating his or her purpose and passion. Focusing positive emotion and moral commitment on the corporal and cognitive acts of care offset, at least to some degree, the very real burdens of caring. The quality of the relationship and the qualities of the self can be strengthened, although things can work the other way, too, weakening both the self and close relationships. It is never only one or the other anyway, but a combination of both—strengthening and weakening—that changes with time, clinical conditions, and personal circumstances.

A person matures as he or she endures both bad times and good times. Without necessarily realizing that things are changing, sometimes deep within the most intimate self, a moral-emotional form of the self evolves. We can just as honestly call it the soul as we can assign it any technical psychological or psychiatric term. The soul is who we are in an existential sense of what we mean to ourselves and others, what we stand for, what we do. Caring involves work on the soul: that of the caregiver and also the receiver of care. This is what I have alluded to as cultivation of the self and of one's relationships. Cultivation, here, represents work. And that work, so much of which is focused on another person, feeds back to engage and readjust who we are. At best it elevates and refines us; at worst it depletes and burdens us. Like yin and yang, augmenting and diminishing are complementary opposites that run together in the human experiences of care.

In my case, I feel as if I replaced, at least partially, who I was in the past with what Joan had become for me. I didn't, I couldn't actually become Joan; yet her caring became part of who I am through the hard and unfinished work of caregiving. I found my soul in that frustrating and elevating work. That the soul I discovered or remade—both seem true—is damaged and scarred seems to me evidence that caregiving is an imperfect project. However great our aspiration for clear, once-and-for-all victory, we are all enmeshed in fragile human conditions that are shot through with failure and inadequacy as much as with hope and achievement—that is the multifaceted and unwieldy reality of living a human life.

The anthropologist in me wants to argue that caregiving is one of the crucial means by which humans have adapted over tens of thousands of years to a cold and impersonal natural world replete with both dangers and opportunities. And it is also how we have sustained and developed societies in response to the very real threats of social suffering and historical change. Seen this way, caring and caregiving give birth to love and redemption but also to regret and inadequacy brought on by our failure to care perfectly. In this nonhumanistic vision, care is ethically neutral, a personal and social process of coping and adapting.

But while it's reasonable to interpret the long evolutionary journey of human beings in this social-science context, it is not, in my experience, the most useful framework for considering the moral and emotional entanglement that characterizes our lives at any given time in the real world. Ethnography provides a different perspective. Care is not just a tool for getting through life by helping one another. It is also a necessary condition for living a life of purpose and passion. Seen this way, caring, and its offspring, love, is a requisite for creating meaning, the most fundamental of human activities. Caring is what is morally and emotionally most at stake in human experience. It is what makes life worth living; it is a source of beauty and goodness. Caring is the embodiment of virtue, the symbolic and material bridge between wisdom and life. And in the face of a world that so easily induces ambiguity and ambivalence, care is one of those few precious things that require authentic commitment and direct action. The arc of history, if it is to bend toward care, must be bent by all of us. Why not start with you and me?

Epilogue

Three years after Joan's death, a young postdoctoral fellow from another university came to ask my advice about an academic project. It was a meeting I didn't really want to take. I had other commitments at that time. I also knew from what I had learned from a brief telephone conversation that my area of specialization did not match up well with the student's plan. I entered the conversation with the idea of making a quick exit. There was something in his voice, however, a hint of anguish, that broke through my natural impatience. I felt a pang of sympathy and sensed there was something at issue that went beyond his academic work. I cannot imagine my younger self picking up on something like this, at least outside of a clinical setting, as my academic persona was always so highly focused on the task at hand.

Even if I had noticed that undercurrent of disquiet, I can't see myself, in the midst of a busy work day with a fixed schedule, taking the time to ask about it. I wouldn't have thought there was time, because I would have been frenetically rushing ahead to the next thing. I wouldn't have regarded this person, a stranger whom I knew not at all, as deserving of the kind of attention I paid to patients or to people in my life to whom I was close. But now I asked. The answer came rushing out like a torrent. It turned out the young man had taken on the burden of care for an older, disabled friend without thinking of the consequences, and he had become exhausted and distraught in the process. He hadn't intended to bear this responsibility beyond the acute phase of his friend's illness. Now he felt trapped by the unwanted and apparently interminable commitment, paralyzed with no idea how to end it. At his wits' end, he spun the story to include his family history and innermost emotional divisions. We stayed together for a long time, talking, listening, working through this difficult experience. I knew that the exchange was important for him, and of course it had resonance for me as well. As we talked, I felt time slow down, my attention intensify, and my presence being drawn out of me.

His feeling of loneliness recalled the feeling I felt at times caring for a greatly diminished Joan. His ambivalence about the caregiving relationship was not at all the dominant feeling I had had caring for Joan, but still I recognized it from my own experiences. He felt coerced to care by the early commitment he had made and by the obligation he now felt. That psychological compulsion had deep roots, deeper than I could explore at the time, but I let him say what he had to say. He thanked me for hearing him out, which had helped him to clarify his difficult situation. I referred him to a professional colleague I respected to further explore this painful relationship and deal with the inner conflict it had generated. Much of what he said stayed with me, though, echoing in the chambers of my memories. There it connected with my thoughts about caring for memories with which I am now always engaged.

There is this existential thing about caregiving: if you allow it to take you over, you find within yourself a tender mercy and a need to act on it. You do what you can, and your very actions put you in the life of another with his or her needs. You cannot respond this way all the time, but that is not really the issue, is it? The genuine question is whether you can find it in yourself to respond with care some of the time, or at bottom, any time. Can you tolerate the pain of another as it enters you and finds your own pain? Memories flow. Caring for that person becomes part of caring for yourself. Remarkably, in some unsought and unexpected way, you end up rebuilding yourself. So when I walked away from this interview, which reprised what I had experienced hundreds of times before, and which had upended my plans for that day, I felt uplifted and less broken.

And I felt the circle being completed. Everything I said and did in this encounter, I learned from Joan: from who she was as a human being, from her care for me, and from the carer she helped me to become. Perhaps that is the bittersweet mystery at the core of care, the soul of care. We are here to care. Yet care is our doubt, our anxiety. It doesn't tie up neatly, if at all, at the end. Inconvenient; often something we would rather not do; at times truly unpleasant; sometimes taking more than it gives; something that can break us. It is also among the most important things we can do. It starts out about others, but in the end it is about us. By giving care, we recognize that we, too, need to be cared for. And that innermost need, our existential precariousness, is also contradicted and made less threatening and more livable by our commitment to another, together with whom we travel toward our shared human end. Perhaps in the end, this is what transforms the soul of care into the care of the soul.

Writing this book, which has preoccupied me for so long, has translated the caring for memories of Joan into caring for me. I have kept Joan alive by taking care of her persona as I adapted it for my own way of being in our strange and troubled time. I also realize now that in one sense I am letting go of Joan by completing a long-drawn-out grieving process with this living testimonial. And in another, equally uncanny sense, the writing has enabled me to allow my old self to slip away, and to be replaced by the author of a book, this book, who is not only a carer of memories, but decidedly a different human being.

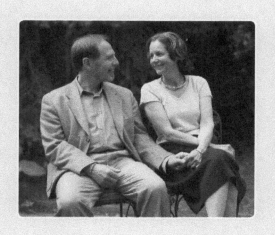

ACKNOWLEDGMENTS

This book emerges from a decade of experience as a primary family caregiver, but it is a lifetime in the making. It brings together almost everything in my personal, academic, and clinical life. It is as much a story of my development as a man and as a doctor as an account of my family and my work. Thousands of hours of conversations, observations, caregiving practices, readings, racking my brain, and the struggle to find words for what I need to say are distilled here. For this reason it is simply impossible to thank the many, many individuals who have helped me, and the families, hospitals, clinics, and nursing homes where I have worked. Or the universities, conferences, and other settings where I have presented my ideas about care and engaged in illuminating colloquiums. But I acknowledge here the vital importance of these experiences to this book.

There would have been no book at all without Joan, and also Anne, Peter, Thomas, Kelly, my grandchildren, my late mother, Marcia, brother Steve, sister-in-law Lee, cousin Laura, and partner Jan. I cannot overstate the valuable help given to Joan and me by our home health aide, to whom I have given the pseudonym Sheilah. I am deeply grateful for all of her assistance.

What I wrote in draft after draft became clarified through the early and fine conceptual editing of Peter Ginna. The later development of the book benefited greatly from an extraordinary editor, David Sobel, who understands from serious experiences what care is about and practices it in his work. My thanks to Peter and David extends to Anne and Jan for their editing. My agent, Jill Kneerim, drew out of me what music is left within, kept the flame going over the years, and represents to me my ideal reader. Kathryn Court at Penguin insisted that showing means more than telling. Victoria Savanh shepherded the book through the production process with care. I've tried to follow the helpful recommendations; where I have fallen short, the failing is mine alone.

A generation of Harvard graduate student research assistants gave me the most practical support. Many Harvard undergraduates and medical students brought their critically minded focus to the inchoate ideas I introduced into my teaching and withstood them with good humor while I worked them out. Postdoctoral fellows and PhD students showed me that mentoring is a caring reciprocity, and that the content and scope of care is always an open question.

My deep thanks to Linda Thomas, my superb assistant, for her enormous contribution to get my longhand, functionally unintelligible scrawl—it is still the only way I can think and write—into the computer files, for offering incisive but modestly proffered advice on all manner of matters and manuscripts, and for keeping me going when my spirit flagged. And before her, Marilyn Goodrich did the same work, also with grace and effectiveness. Claire de Forcrand helped assemble materials for the final manuscript.

My great debt goes to the thousands of patients, family members, and health professionals with whom I have had the remarkable privilege to work over half a century in the United

States, China, Taiwan, Japan, the Philippines, the United Kingdom, Kenya, Tanzania, South Africa, and elsewhere in the world. Whatever wisdom I have managed to grasp and express on caregiving comes from them.

The long-term benefactor of Harvard's Medical Anthropology Program was the late Michael Crichton. He created the fund that, among many other things, supported the writing of this book. I hope I have honored the only charge he gave me—"to always go against the grain of medicine." Over the decades the research I have drawn upon for *The Soul of Care* was funded by many sources, including the National Institutes of Health, the National Science Foundation, the Rockefeller Foundation, the MacArthur Foundation, the Carnegie Corporation, the Freeman Foundation, the Social Science Research Council, and the Guggenheim Foundation, among others. I remain deeply grateful for this support.

I have been a member of Harvard University for over four decades, where the Department of Anthropology in the Faculty of Arts and Sciences and the Department of Global Health and Social Medicine in Harvard Medical School have been my home. I owe a deep debt of gratitude to my colleagues in both departments, and an even greater debt to the university as a whole. Harvard provided nursing care for Joan in her last year of working with me so that she could stay in our offices, where I could watch and assist her and still carry out my teaching responsibilities. Harvard supported my career-long interests, providing me with great collaborators and superb students. And Harvard also gave me the very special gift of time and space and resources to build a program in medical anthropology with care at its very center. This book is only the latest of that program's accomplishments.

Finally, an honest admission. *The Soul of Care* is not yet finished. I could keep writing it over and over and still not finish. (In fact,

I am even a little frightened to come to an end, and wonder, What comes next?) This is because the subject remains alive and continues to resist my struggle to wrestle it into words that are adequate and telling. Care is like life itself—incomplete and unfinishable. But perhaps my efforts in these pages will contribute to the building of a moral movement for care where others will pick up the torch and realize more fully its significance for us all.

Arthur Kleinman
Cambridge, Massachusetts
South Bristol, Maine
and Rozelle, NSW, Australia

WORKS CITED AND FOR FURTHER READING

Abel, Emily K. *The Inevitable Hour: A History of Caring for Dying Patients in America*. Baltimore: Johns Hopkins University Press, 2016.

Abraham, Laurie Kaye. *Mama Might Be Better Off Dead: The Failure of Health Care in Urban America*. Chicago: University of Chicago Press, 1994.

Alterra, Aaron [E. S. Goldman]. *The Caregiver: A Life With Alzheimer's*. Hanover, NH: Steerforth Press, 1999.

Bayley, John. *Elegy for Iris*. New York: Picador, 1999.

Bellini, Lisa M., and Judy A. Shea. "Mood Change and Empathy Decline Persist During Three Years of Internal Medicine Training." *Academic Medicine* 80, no. 2 (2005): 164–167.

Biehl, João. *Vita: Life in a Zone of Social Abandonment*. Berkeley: University of California Press, 2005.

Boris, Eileen, and Jennifer Klein. *Caring for America: Home Health Workers in the Shadow of the Welfare State*. Oxford, UK: Oxford University Press, 2012.

Brodwin, Paul E. *Everyday Ethics: Voices from the Front Line of Community Psychiatry*. Berkeley: University of California Press, 2012.

Buch, Elana D. "Anthropology of Aging and Care." *Annual Review of Anthropology* 44 (2015): 277–293.

Cassidy, Sheila. *Sharing the Darkness: The Spirituality of Caring*. New York: Orbis Books, 1992.

Coakley, Sarah, and Kay Kaufman Shemelay, eds. *Pain and Its Transformations: The Interface of Biology and Culture*. Cambridge, MA: Harvard University Press, 2008.

Culture, Medicine, and Psychiatry: An International Journal of Cross-Cultural Health Research. New York: Springer US.

Das, Veena. *Affliction: Health, Disease, Poverty.* New York: Fordham University Press, 2015.

Didion, Joan. *The Year of Magical Thinking.* New York: Alfred A. Knopf, 2005.

Fadiman, Anne. *The Spirit Catches You and You Fall Down: A Hmong Child, Her American Doctors, and the Collision of Two Cultures.* New York: Farrar, Straus and Giroux, 2012.

Farmer, Paul, Arthur Kleinman, Jim Kim, and Matthew Basilico, eds. *Reimagining Global Health: An Introduction.* Berkeley: University of California Press, 2013.

Foner, Nancy. *The Caregiving Dilemma: Work in an American Nursing Home.* Berkeley: University of California Press, 1994.

Foucault, Michel. *Discipline and Punishment. The Birth of the Prison.* Translated by Alan Sheridan. London: Allen Lang, 1977.

Frankl, Viktor. *Man's Search for Meaning.* Boston: Beacon Press, 2006 [1946].

Fry, Erika, and Fred Schulte. "Death by a Thousand Clicks." *Fortune*, March 18, 2019.

Fuchs, Elinor. *Making an Exit: A Mother-Daughter Drama with Alzheimer's, Machine Tools, and Laughter.* New York: Metropolitan Books, 2005.

Garcia, Angela. *The Pastoral Clinic: Addiction and Dispossession along the Rio Grande.* Berkeley: University of California Press, 2010.

Gawande, Atul. *Being Mortal: Medicine and What Matters in the End.* New York: Picador, 2015.

———. "The Upgrade: Why Doctors Hate Their Computers." *New Yorker* 94, no. 36 (2018): 62.

Geertz, Clifford. *Local Knowledge.* New York: Basic Books, 1987.

Glenn, Evelyn Nakano. *Forced to Care: Coercion and Caregiving in America.* Cambridge, MA: Harvard University Press, 2012.

Good, Byron. *Medicine, Rationality, and Experience: An Anthropological Perspective.* Cambridge, UK: Cambridge University Press, 1994.

Good, Mary-Jo DelVecchio. *American Medicine: The Quest for Competence.* Berkeley: University of California Press, 1995.

Grant, Karen R., Carol Amaratunga, Pat Armstrong, Madeline Boscoe, Ann Pederson, and Kay Wilson, eds. *Caring For/Caring About: Women, Home Care, and Unpaid Caregiving.* Toronto: University of Toronto Press, 2004.

Groopman, Jerome E. *The Measure of Our Days: A Spiritual Exploration of Illness.* New York: Penguin, 1998.

Gross, Jane. *A Bittersweet Season: Caring for Our Aging Parents—and Ourselves.* New York: Alfred A. Knopf, 2011.

Hampton, J. R, M. J. Harrison, J. R. Mitchell, J. S. Prichard, and C. Seymour. "Relative Contributions of History-Taking, Physical Examination, and Laboratory Investigation to Diagnosis and Management of Medical Outpatients." *British Medical Journal* 2 (1975): 486.

Heaney, Seamus, *Opened Ground: Poems, 1966–1996.* London: Faber and Faber, 1998.

Hojat, Mohammadreza, Salvatore Mangione, Thomas J. Nasca, Susan Rattner, James B. Erdmann, Joseph S. Gonnella, and Mike Magee. "An Empirical Study of Decline in Empathy in Medical School." *Medical Education* 38, no. 9 (2004): 934–941.

Institute of Medicine Committee on Pain, Disability, and Chronic Illness Behavior. Marian Osterweis, Arthur Kleinman, and David Mechanic, eds. *Pain and Disability: Clinical, Behavioral, and Public Policy Perspectives.* Washington, DC: National Academies Press, 1987.

Jackson, Stanley W. "Presidential Address: The Wounded Healer." *Bulletin of the History of Medicine* 75, no. 1 (2001): 1–36.

Jamison, Kay Redfield. *An Unquiet Mind: A Memoir of Moods and Madness.* New York: Vintage Books, 1996.

Kalanithi, Paul. *When Breath Becomes Air.* New York: Random House, 2016.

Kaptchuk, Ted. "The Placebo Effect in Alternative Medicine: Can the Performance of a Healing Ritual Have Clinical Significance?" *Annals of Internal Medicine* 136, no. 11 (2002): 817–825.

Kaptchuk, Ted J., and Franklin G. Miller. "Placebo Effects in Medicine." *New England Journal of Medicine* 373, no. 1 (2015): 8–9.

Kaufman, Sharon R. *And a Time to Die: How American Hospitals Shape the End of Life.* New York: Scribner, 2005.

Kleinman, Arthur. *Patients and Healers in the Context of Culture: An Exploration of the Borderland between Anthropology, Medicine, and Psychiatry.* Berkeley: University of California Press, 1980.

———. *Social Origins of Distress and Disease: Depression, Neurasthenia, and Pain in Modern China.* New Haven, CT: Yale University Press, 1986.

———. *The Illness Narratives.* New York: Basic Books, 1988.

———. *What Really Matters: Living a Moral Life amidst Uncertainty and Danger.* Oxford: Oxford, UK: University Press, 2007.

———. "Catastrophe and Caregiving: The Failure of Medicine as an Art." *Lancet* 371, no. 9606 (2008): 22–23.

———. "Caregiving: The Odyssey of Becoming More Human." *Lancet* 373, no. 9660 (2009): 292–293.

———. "Caregiving as Moral Experience." *Lancet* 380, no. 9853 (2012): 1550–1551.

———. "From Illness as Culture to Caregiving as Moral Experience." *New England Journal of Medicine* 368 (2013): 1376–1377.

———. "Caring for Memories." *Lancet* 387, no. 10038 (2016): 2596–2597.

———. "Presence." *Lancet* 389, no. 10088 (2017): 2466–2467.

Kleinman, Arthur, and Joan Kleinman. "How Bodies Remember: Social Memory and Bodily Experience of Criticism, Resistance, and Delegitimation following China's Cultural Revolution." *New Literary History* 25, no. 3 (1994): 707–723.

———. "The Appeal of Experience; The Dismay of Images: Cultural Appropriations of Suffering in Our Times." *Daedalus* 125, no. 1 (1996): 1–23.

Kleinman, Arthur, Yunxiang Yan, Jing Jun, Sing Lee, Everett Zhang, Pan Tianshu, Wu Fei, and Jinhua Guo. *Deep China: The Moral Life of the Person.* Berkeley: University of California Press, 2011.

Kuhn, Thomas. *The Structure of Scientific Revolutions.* Chicago: University of Chicago Press, 1970 [1962].

Lasch, Christopher. *Haven in a Heartless World: The Family Besieged.* New York: W. W. Norton, 1995.

Levitsky, Sandra R. *Caring for Our Own: Why There Is No Political Demand for New American Social Welfare Rights.* New York: Oxford University Press, 2014.

Lewis-Fernández, Roberto, and Naelys Díaz. "The Cultural Formulation: A Method for Assessing Cultural Factors Affecting the Clinical Encounter." *Psychiatric Quarterly* 73, no. 4 (2002): 271–295.

Mattingly, Cheryl. *Healing Dramas and Clinical Plots: The Narrative Structure of Experience.* Cambridge, UK; New York: Cambridge University Press, 1998.

Mda, Zakes. *Ways of Dying.* New York: Picador, 2002.

Mechanic, David, Donna D. McAlpine, and Marsha Rosenthal. "Are Patients' Office Visits with Physicians Getting Shorter?" *New England Journal of Medicine* 344 (2001): 198–204.

Merton, Robert K. "The Unanticipated Consequences of Purposive Social Action." *American Sociological Review* 1, no. 6 (1936): 894–904.

Miles, Ann. *Living with Lupus: Women and Chronic Illness in Ecuador.* Austin: University of Texas Press, 2013.

Mol, Annemarie. *The Logic of Care: Health and the Problem of Patient Choice.* New York: Routledge, 2008.

Morris, David B. *The Culture of Pain.* Berkeley: University of California Press, 1993.

Mukherjee, Siddhartha. *The Emperor of All Maladies: A Biography of Cancer.* New York: Simon & Schuster, 2010.

Mulley, Albert G., Chris Trimble, and Glyn Elwyn. "Stop the Silent Misdiagnosis: Patients' Preferences Matter." *British Medical Journal* 345 (2012): e6572.

National Academies of Sciences, Engineering, and Medicine. Richard Schulz and Jill Eden, eds. *Families Caring for an Aging America.* Washington, DC: National Academies Press, 2016.

Nelson, Sioban, and Suzanne Gordon, eds. *The Complexities of Care: Nursing Reconsidered.* Ithaca, NY: ILR Press/Cornell University Press, 2006.

Nightingale, Florence. *Notes on Nursing: What It Is, and What It Is Not.* New York: Appleton, 1860.

Ofri, Danielle. *What Patients Say, What Doctors Hear.* Boston: Beacon Press, 2017.

O'Reilly, Dermot, Michael Rosato, and Aideen Maguire. "Caregiving Reduces Mortality Risk for Most Caregivers: A Census-Based Record Linkage Study." *International Journal of Epidemiology* 44, no. 6 (2015): 1959–1969.

Osterman, Paul. *Who Will Care for Us? Long-Term Care and the Long-Term Workforce.* New York: Russell Sage Foundation, 2017.

Patel, Vikram, Harry Minas, Alex Cohen, and Martin J. Prince, eds. *Global Mental Health: Principles and Practice.* Oxford, UK: Oxford University Press, 2013.

Peckins, Christopher S., Leila R. Khorashadi, and Edward Wolpow. "A Case of Reduplicative Paramnesia for Home." *Cognitive and Behavioral Neurology* 29, no. 3 (2016): 150–157.

Poo, Ai-jen, and Ariane Conrad. *The Age of Dignity: Preparing for the Elder Boom in a Changing America.* New York: New Press, 2015.

Puett, Michael, and Christine Gross-Loh. *The Path: What Chinese Philosophers Can Teach Us About the Good Life.* New York: Simon & Schuster, 2017. First published 2016.

Richardson, Robert D. *William James: In the Maelstrom of American Modernism.* Boston: Houghton Mifflin Harcourt, 2006.

Sankar, Andrea. *Dying at Home: A Family Guide for Caregiving.* Baltimore: Johns Hopkins University Press, 1991.

Sherr Klein, Bonnie. *Slow Dance: A Story of Stroke, Love and Disability.* Toronto: Vintage Canada, 1997.

Simmons, Philip. *Learning to Fall: The Blessings of an Imperfect Life.* New York: Bantam Books, 2003.

Slaughter, Anne-Marie. *Unfinished Business: Women Men Work Family.* New York: Random House, 2015.

Solomon, Andrew. *The Noonday Demon: An Atlas of Depression.* New York: Scribner, 2014.

Stevenson, Lisa. *Life Beside Itself: Imagining Care in the Canadian Arctic.* Berkeley: University of California Press, 2014.

Swift, Jonathan. *A Modest Proposal for Preventing the Children of Poor People from being a Burthen to their Parents or Country, and for Making them Beneficial to the Publick.* Dublin: S. Harding; London: J. Roberts, 1729.

Taylor, Janelle S. "On Recognition, Caring, and Dementia." *Medical Anthropology Quarterly* 22, no. 4 (2008): 313–335.

Tronto, Joan. *Moral Boundaries: A Political Argument for an Ethic of Care.* New York: Routledge, 1993.

———. *Caring Democracy: Markets, Equality, and Justice.* New York: New York University Press, 2013.

Verghese, Abraham. *My Own Country: A Doctor's Story.* New York: Vintage Books, 1995.

Weiming, Tu, and Mary Evelyn Tucker, eds. *Confucian Spirituality.* Spring Valley, NY: Crossroad, 2003.

Witchel, Alex. *All Gone: A Memoir of My Mother's Dementia.* New York: Riverhead Books, 2012.

Wood, Diana F. "Bullying and Harassment in Medical Schools: Still Rife and Must Be Tackled." *British Medical Journal* 333, no. 7570 (2006): 664–665.